The Healing Machi

Series: Epistemologies of Healing
General Editors: David Parkin and Elisabeth Hsu: University of Oxford

This series publishes monographs and edited volumes on Indigenous (so-called traditional) medical knowledge and practice, alternative and complementary medicine, and ethnobiological studies that relate to health and illness. The emphasis of the series is on the way Indigenous epistemologies inform healing, against a background of comparison with other practices, and in recognition of the fluidity between them.

Recent volumes:

Volume 23
The Healing Machi: An Ethnography of Mapuche Medicine Efficacies
Adelaida Barros

Volume 22
Fragile Futures: Ambiguities of Care in Burkina Faso
Helle Samuelsen

Volume 21
Breathing Hearts: Sufism, Healing, and Anti-Muslim Racism in Germany
Nasima Selim

Volume 20
Chinese Medicine in East Africa: An Intimacy with Strangers
Elisabeth Hsu

Volume 19
Configuring Contagion: Ethnographies of Biosocial Epidemics
Edited by Lotte Meinert and Jens Seeberg

Volume 18
Fierce Medicines, Fragile Socialities: Grounding Global HIV Treatment in Tanzania
Dominik Mattes

Volume 17
Capturing Quicksilver: The Position, Power, and Plasticity of Chinese Medicine in Singapore
Arielle A. Smith

Volume 16
Ritual Retellings: Luangan Healing Performances through Practice
Isabell Herrmans

Volume 15
Healing Roots: Anthropology in Life and Medicine
Julie Laplante

Volume 14
Asymmetrical Conversations: Contestations, Circumventions, and the Blurring of Therapeutic Boundaries
Edited by Harish Naraindas, Johannes Quack, and William S. Sax

Volume 13
The Body in Balance: Humoral Medicines in Practice
Edited by Peregrine Horden and Elisabeth Hsu

For a full volume listing, please see the series page on our website:
https://www.berghahnbooks.com/series/epistemologies-of-healing

The Healing Machi

An Ethnography of Mapuche Medicine Efficacies

Adelaida Barros

berghahn
NEW YORK • OXFORD
www.berghahnbooks.com

First published in 2026 by
Berghahn Books
www.berghahnbooks.com

Library of Congress Cataloging-in-Publication Data
A C.I.P. cataloging record is available from the Library of Congress
Library of Congress Cataloging in Publication Control Number: 2026032642

British Library Cataloguing in Publication Data
A catalogue record for this book is available from the British Library

EU GPSR Authorized Representative
LOGOS EUROPE, 9 rue Nicolas Poussin, 17000, LA ROCHELLE, France
Email: Contact@logoseurope.eu

ISBN 978-1-80758-022-3 hardback
ISBN 978-1-80758-023-0 epub
ISBN 978-1-80758-024-7 web pdf

https://doi.org/10.3167/9781807580223

Contents

Introduction

I met Miguel on a September afternoon in a café in downtown Santiago.[1] A friend in common put us in contact. I was hoping Miguel could help me to find gatekeepers and key informants in my intent to enter the field in the Araucanía region, 500 miles south of Santiago. Miguel was a doctor in his early forties who, at the time I met him, was working as a radiologist in a public hospital in the northern area of Santiago. Miguel's father was born in a Mapuche rural community in Puaucho, Araucanía. Like many other Mapuche throughout the twentieth century, Miguel's father migrated to the capital in search of better job opportunities. Like most Mapuche today, Miguel was born in Santiago, far away from where his paternal family was originally from.

Miguel started the conversation by explaining that he was *awingkado* (Westernized) and, thus, did not think he could be of much help for my research. I had to look for people who really knew about Mapuche spirituality and medicine, Miguel suggested. He went on to explain that among urban Mapuche migrants, an Indigenous identity used to be a source of shame and discrimination. Therefore, his father did not speak to his sons in Mapudungun, the Mapuche language, and did not teach them anything about Mapuche culture. Quite the opposite, his father tried to conceal the fact that he was Mapuche. Later, I heard numerous similar stories both among urban and rural Mapuche. Parents and grandparents tried to protect their children from discrimination by not teaching them the language or any other aspect of Mapuche culture and, thus, concealing their identity. Unlike his father, Miguel said he was not ashamed of being Mapuche. In fact, he stated that it was a pity his father, now deceased, did not teach him Mapudungun. He wished he could speak it. He had even tried to learn a bit. Miguel thought it was sad that Mapuche knowledge had ceased to be transmitted from parents to children, adding that he had friends who were Mapuche descendants and were trying to learn Mapudungun and become engaged in Mapuche ritual life and spirituality. These friends were not raised as Mapuche but were now trying to "know more about their culture," as Miguel put it.

Miguel was amused by my interest in Mapuche medicine. He thought it was unusual for a doctor like me because most doctors discard Mapuche medicine as superstition or just placebo. In fact, like any other doctor, Miguel was skeptical regarding the efficacy of Mapuche medicine. He confided in me that he once went to see a machi, or a Mapuche shaman, because he was experiencing a skin rash. This occurred on one of his regular trips to visit his aunt, his father's youngest sister, in Puaucho, Araucanía. Miguel's aunt took him to the local state-sponsored Mapuche medical center. There, Miguel received *lawen* (remedies) from a machi in the form of medicinal herbal infusions. He laughed when stating that the remedy did not have any effect. Miguel thought his rash was due to stress and, therefore, psychological support probably made more sense to him as treatment. Miguel's skepticism was something I expected. However, what he said next was unexpected: "But not all machi are real machi, you need to be careful with machi, you need to know the right people who can tell you who to talk to." A "real" machi, I learned, was someone with the spiritual gift (Spanish: *don*) to heal. This gift is obtained through a machi's *pülli* (lineage spirit). Therefore, people who become machi because they were trained or went to a machi school were fake machi: they do not have a spiritual gift. Miguel thought that, perhaps, he had not been healed because the machi who treated him was not a real machi. Also, he suggested I needed to know the right people who could recommend a real machi to me; that is, people who have already been treated satisfactorily by a machi, or people with more experience of dealing with machi.

In retrospect, my first encounter with a Mapuche person already contained the two elements at the heart of this ethnography. The first one was driven by my own theoretical preoccupations regarding medical efficacy and was elicited due to the questions I asked and the themes I wanted to talk about. Miguel also wanted to talk about the efficacy of Mapuche medicine, and he phrased this concern, for the first time, as many friends did later: some machi are real and some machi are not. Some machi can cure ill people while others are just pretending. The second element Miguel put forward was not elicited by my questions. Rather, I encountered it recurrently throughout a twelve-month period of fieldwork. Miguel introduced me to a narrative based on feelings of loss and nostalgia regarding a Mapuche culture that was never taught to him and, thus, he did not know. Feelings of loss and dispossession and the necessity to recover what was lost were a core theme among my Mapuche interlocutors.

Methodological Considerations

This book is based on a doctoral thesis in Social Anthropology at the University of Oxford. The research presented here was funded by the Government of Chile through the state agency ANID (Agencia Nacional de Investigación y Desarrollo). This ethnography is the product of a twelve-month period of fieldwork mostly in the coastal area of the Araucanía region, between September 2016 and September 2017. However, a strict delimitation of a geographical field site would be misleading. This is so because machi usually travel long distances to treat patients, and patients also travel long distances to seek the help of a machi. At the same time, the distinction between urban and rural is blurred, since people continuously move from rural communities to towns and cities (and vice versa). The continuity of rural and urban spaces, in the Mapuche context, has already been described by other authors (e.g., Bacigalupo 2007; Bengoa and Caniguan 2012). Therefore, although most observations presented here happened in rural areas, some occurred in towns and cities.

I entered the field in Araucanía through two different entry points. The first entry point was through scholars in the Intercultural and Indigenous Studies Centre (Centro de Estudios Interculturales e Indígenas) at the Institute of Sociology of the Catholic University of Chile, whom I contacted in Santiago. Through these scholars, I was able to meet other scholars on the Catholic University campus in Villarrica, a town located east of Temuco, in Araucanía. Once in Villarrica, and while being housed by the local campus of the Catholic University, scholars there introduced me to the Mapuche team working in a state-funded Mapuche medical center. The Mapuche medical center was located west of Temuco, near the coast. I was also introduced to someone who later became my Mapudungun teacher and provided significant insight into Mapuche medicine throughout my fieldwork. My Mapudungun teacher used to collaborate with scholars at the Catholic University on different projects and lived in a rural area near Lake Budi.

After being introduced to the medical team working in a state-funded medical center, I explained my research project to them, and they accepted my presence as an ethnographer at their workplace. Thus, I moved from Villarrica, in the mountains, to the coast. I conducted a three-month ethnography in the Mapuche medical center while renting a room in a house in the local town. During that period, I spent every day, from Monday to Friday, and from 8 a.m. to 5 p.m., at the medical center. However, this is not a hospital ethnography. Rather, I strategically used the medical center to generate relationships with key people and machi. Later, I moved from the medical center to the communities. Thus, most of the observations provided here describe medical practices carried out at private homes and communities.

My second entry point was through my friend, Miguel, whom I already mentioned. Miguel put me in contact with his family in the south. In fact, in the first meeting we had, he called his aunt, Amelia, so I could talk to her and ask her whether I could stay at her place. Amelia was a widow who lived with her two teenage daughters, and she became a dear friend. Amelia and her family introduced me to neighbors and the extended family, with whom I spent plenty of family and social occasions. Throughout a year of fieldwork, I spent a couple of days at Amelia's place in Puaucho at regular intervals of about two or three weeks.

Fieldwork methods included participant observation, language learning (together with weekly lessons at my teacher's home; I took a 24-hour course on basic Mapudungun at the Catholic University of Temuco) and the study of the literature written on the Mapuche from colonial times to the present day. Although I initially conducted some semi-structured interviews, which were recorded, I quickly discovered that it was more fruitful to engage in informal conversations. This was so because people talked more freely, and were easier to engage in informal conversations rather than recorded semi-structured interviews. Therefore, most of the observations presented here derive from unstructured, but persistent and immersive participant observation.

I closely observed the work of three female machi with whom I spent a considerable amount of time in their homes and communities. I also traveled with one of them to attend to patients in various areas of the Araucanía, Los Lagos and Aysén regions. I repeatedly observed the work of another three machi (one female and two male) because I was accompanying friends who were sick or because I was invited to a community ceremony or to a ritual healing event. In addition, I met two female *machil* (machi initiates).

The Focus of this Ethnography

The main purpose of this ethnography is to provide a rationale for positive experiential transformations (or lack of them) in the context of Mapuche ritual healing, from the perspective of the phenomenology of the body. I intend to give both an ethnographic account of what counts as positive healing transformations in the Mapuche context and to theoretically contribute to the discussion of ritual healing efficacy from a phenomenological perspective.

This ethnography examines how people know who is a real machi or a Mapuche shaman. Or in other words, who can really know, treat and prevent illnesses and misfortunes. This question, which preoccupied my interlocutors, is different to that of why a machi is popular or has a lot of clients. The popularity of a machi can be influenced by issues of power and status, such as wealth and ties with the local government; personality, such as charisma, empathy and self-confidence; family and community support; and, also, the skills and knowledge to exert positive healing transformations. The question of who is a real machi is also different to the question of authenticity, understood in terms of historical veracity and genuine traditions. Here, my main concern, and that of my interlocutors, is what defines a real machi in terms of their skills to use transformative techniques in the context of curative and preventive ritual healing. Admittedly, I cannot completely separate this question from the issue of popularity and authenticity (neither do my Mapuche interlocutors). However, focusing on transformative techniques and skills does imply an emphasis on bodily transformations when discussing medical efficacy. Thus, the question of who is a real machi is fundamentally an existential question touching on issues of what being healed (or transformed) through ritual action is.

I explore two main characteristics that, according to my Mapuche interlocutors, make a machi a real machi. First, a real machi must have the spiritual gift to "see" the illness or problem through different divinatory techniques. The spiritual ability to see is obtained through a *pülli* (lineage spirit), which differentiates machi from people who learn to be or are trained as healers. Therefore, I explore how it is that a machi can see, and different ways of seeing. In other words, how a machi can know an illness or problem and treat it. Secondly, a real machi has *kimün* (ancestral knowledge) regarding the Mapuche lifeworld. Significantly, machi achieve *kimün* not only through learning from elders, but also through *peuma* (dreams) and *küymin* (ritual trance). Machi are the only type of person who can experience *küymin*, a state in which a machi is possessed by their *pülli* who can, then, deliver a spiritual message. Thus, a machi is indispensable for the transmission of *kimün* and the continuity of Mapuche ritual life and spirituality. To do so, machi preside over traditional ceremonies that aim to prevent illnesses and misfortunes and maintain the lifestyle of the group. Therefore, being a real machi means both divining and treating illnesses and misfortunes effectively and presiding over traditional ceremonies effectively. In this way, machi have a role both as healers and as knowledge and community builders.

To address the second characteristic of a real machi, that of a person with *kimün* (ancestral knowledge) responsible for community building and transmission of cultural practices and knowledge, a phenomenological approach needs to be complemented. Ritual healing transformations not only have an existential function, but they also have a political function. Therefore, this work combines a phenomenological approach with careful attention to the social and political context. Specifically, this ethnography seeks to link healing rituals and individual bodily transformations with the politics of Mapuche identity. In that spirit, I deliberately begin this ethnography in Santiago, miles away from the area in which I conducted fieldwork, and with a conversation with a Mapuche doctor who thought he did not know enough about Mapuche medicine. In this manner, I try to do justice to a story of dispossession of land, knowledge and cultural practices that many friends, such as Miguel, were eager to talk about. Thus, this work attends to the role of machi and medical practices in generating and controlling both a collective Mapuche identity and a personal Mapuche identity based on shared feelings of pride and self-esteem.

The Problem of Medical Efficacy from a Phenomenological Perspective

My ethnographic exploration of how to know who is a real machi in the Mapuche context is related to broader anthropological preoccupations; namely, the problem of the efficacy of the so-called traditional medical practices. Although some have argued (e.g., Waldram 2000) that medical anthropology initially neglected the problem of efficacy, assuming that ritual healing and traditional medical practices inevitably produce socially predictable outcomes, this is not the case within the field of medical anthropology today. Efficacy has been widely problematized, but one should recognize that efficacy is not one single thing: medical efficacy can be defined in multiple ways. Efficacy, then, is plural, and multiple efficacies are not mutually exclusive. Here, following Csordas (1994a), I understand efficacy as ritually induced transformations of the self. The term "ritual" is significant since it denotes that healing transformations occur in a socially and technically demarcated time and space, from which ritual action reorganizes experience and has the potential to transform a problematic situation (Hsu 2015; Kapferer 2004; Lewis 1980). In addition, the self is proposed to be understood as the object of transformation of ritual healing (Csordas 1994a). The self is understood not only as a person with a defined set of characteristics, but also as the process of constitution of the person and their world. Csordas (ibid.) refers to processes of constitution of a person and their world as self-processes. Self-processes start in bodily pre-reflexive experience and end in an individualized self: a person with a differentiated set of characteristics. Csordas' proposal is to center attention on ongoing processes of individuation or objectification, rather than starting from the already objectified self.

In this way, Csordas (1994a) emphasizes aspects of self-transformations, which occur at a level that is pre-reflexive or prior to conscious awareness. The use of the terms pre-reflexive/reflexive allows for a non-dichotomist division in which what is pre-reflexive is always accessible to becoming reflexive. Reflexivity refers to the human capacity to make something conscious (or the capacity for objectification). Thus, reflexivity refers to the capacity to cognitively (understood as a deliberative, effortful conscious process) take the self and others as objects, while pre-reflexive experience is pre-objective but available to objectification.

Why is pre-reflexive experience, as the starting point of self-processes, relevant in the Mapuche context? Machi are expected to "see" an illness or a problematic situation through divinatory techniques, such as the visual inspection of a patient's bottled urine. Patients expect proof that the machi can see without them explaining. Here, the sense of vision is understood as having an objectifying and detaching quality. Seeing is also associated with knowing, and patients can only have proof that a machi knows if they name the illness or problem. Thus, seeing is the capacity to know the problematic circumstances of a person without the necessity of explanation, which is made apparent through the machi speech. Divination rituals are rich in pre-reflexive experience such as the direction of attention, the promotion of imagination, and the manipulation of the senses and the emotions. Through the technical elaboration of experience that is immediate (not mediated by deliberative, effortful conscious processing) and embodied, a skillful machi can see an illness or problem and also make it visible to the patient. After seeing, machi and patient can engage in a reflexive understanding of a problematic situation and its possible solutions. Therefore, reflexive understanding is grounded in bodily experience, which is largely pre-reflexive.

In the same vein, machi are expected to make evil spirits visible in the context of ritual action directed at illnesses caused by evil forces. The invisible nature of evil spirits and the incapacity of biomedical testing to visualize them (or to visualizes their negative effects on people's bodies) is the source of their power according to some of my interlocutors. If a machi makes evil spirits visible, then people have proof that evil spirits are indeed the agents of affliction. Moreover, healing action can be directed against evil forces once they have been seen. Machi promote the visualization of evil spirits through different sensory modalities such as vision, sound, touch, and negative emotions such as fear. As in divinatory techniques, ritual actions targeted at evil spirits organize sensory experience and the emotions so that the evil spirit can be objectified and, then, neutralized and disposed of.

Machi are also expected to make benign spirits present or embody the spirits of the ancestors. As stated previously, a machi's ability to experience *küymin* (ritual trance), or the ritually induced possession of a machi by the spirit of a deceased shaman, is important for the continuity and transmission of cultural practices and the Mapuche lifeworld. Through *küymin*, a community of people can communicate with "spirits from the past," which is fundamental in struggles to recover *kimün* (ancestral knowledge) lost in the process of colonization. To make the spirit present through *küymin*, collective ritual action is directed both at the machi's body and the communal body. Dancing, playing music, shouting, and drinking together are bodily skills and acts that make the spirits come. When the spirits are finally present, only after laborious and concerted ritual action can they deliver an important message to the community, usually in the form of a sung prayer on the part of the machi. The message is later discussed and interpreted in conversations during and after a ceremony. The embodiment of the ancestors is fundamental in creating and maintaining a Mapuche way of knowing the past and engaging with the present and the future.

In this manner, both in divinatory techniques, ritual healing directed at evil spirits, and ritual trance, agents of afflictions or spirits from the past are objectified through self-processes. For instance, an evil spirit is visualized in the form of the scream of a child, an illness is revealed in a patient's urine, or an ancestor warns of possible natural disasters if people stop celebrating Mapuche ceremonies. I propose to understand these techniques as directed at self-processes through which objectification of a problematic situation occurs. The process starts in a layer of experience that is immediate and embodied, and upon which a reflexive elaboration of the cause of an illness or a problem and the exploration of possible solutions is built. Thus, the reflexive understanding of an illness or problem and its solutions is grounded in the body and its practices and skills. Stated differently, reflexive elaborations grounded in the body become experientially meaningful through ritual healing acts.

To explore how reflexivity is grounded in the body, I draw on Csordas' (1994a: 74–87) understanding of imagination as a mode of self-process or as a mode of orientation toward the world. Here, imagination is both a form of doing and orienting the body in the world and a way of reflexively engaging with a problematic situation. Stated otherwise, imagination is a human capacity through which self-processes move from indeterminacy to orientation, from the pre-reflexive to reflexive understanding and objectification. Thus, through imagination, the subject can engage with the world and others in meaningful ways. Phenomenologically, imagination is something that the body does, an act (Sartre 2004), or the bodily simulation of possible experiences of imagined objects (Jansen 2018: 686). To imagine something, then, is to relate to that imagined object and not only to a mental image that represents something absent. Thus, imagination, understood as a bodily act, presents an existential situation. At the same time, the content of imagination represents a cultural meaning and, as such, imagination belongs to the order of representation. Csordas proposes the complementarity of the semiotic and the phenomenological understanding of imagination (1994a: 80–81) by claiming that imagination is culturally intelligible since it belongs to the semiotic order, and, also, performatively efficacious as it is a mode of orientation toward the world or the active engagement of the body with its world.

In this way, I follow Csordas' reflections on imagination to postulate a complementarity between symbolic and phenomenological approaches to ritual healing efficacy. Thus, an understanding of efficacy as ritually induced transformations of self-processes does not try to compete with or replace a symbolic understanding of medical efficacy. Rather, my focus on pre-reflexive experience and its relationship with reflexivity is an attempt to ground symbols in the body and, thus, portray how symbolic formations become existentially meaningful. In this way, I can explore the paradox that while Mapuche ritual healing is largely relying on techniques that are nonverbal and embodied, at the same time the final objective of ritual action is knowing or seeing. For example, when consulting a machi, people expect them to produce the correct visualization of an illness in a patient's bottled urine, which is revealed through speech. Or the multisensory and affective experience of collective ritual action aims to make the spirits come, so they can deliver a message to the community. The message is received with careful attention, and later discussions and interpretations of what a spirit said while a machi was in trance occur at the end of a ceremony and continue to develop for some time after a ritual occurrence.

The understanding of the self as a constitutive process occurring every time the subject relates to someone or something that is significant to the study of healing. The self, in this way understood, is susceptible to transformations through treatment. However, self-processes occur under cultural and historical constraints that explain both the continuity of the sense of self and the limits of ritual transformations. Although there is space for transformations to occur, we cannot completely create a novel self regardless of its past and cultural context. To explain these constraints Csordas (1990) turns to Bourdieu's concept of the habitus to complement Merleau-Ponty's phenomenology. In this way, careful attention is placed here on the political context in which the Mapuche engage in acts of healing. Healing actions are embedded in political discourses and practices that are aimed at recovering *kimün* (ancestral knowledge) to create and recreate the *küme mongen* (wellbeing, literally good living) of the Mapuche and their world vis-à-vis the Chileans.

The Mapuche in Chile

The Mapuche are Indigenous peoples of Chile and Argentina. In Chile, 1,623,073 people identified themselves as Mapuche in the last census of 2024, which corresponds to almost 9 percent of the total Chilean population and 76 percent of the Chilean Indigenous population (INE 2025). Most of the Mapuche population today lives in Santiago, which is the consequence of rural-urban migration throughout the twentieth century. However, Araucanía remains the region in Chile with the highest demographic proportion of Mapuche in the country, relative to the general population (23 percent of the total Araucanía population). Araucania is the region in Chile with the highest rate of poverty and rurality and the lowest rate of population growth. Other regions in Chile with an important Mapuche population are Los Lagos and Biobío.

In Araucanía, most Mapuche live in rural areas, in the so-called Indigenous Communities, which are the consequence of war, historical displacement, and land loss. In these communities, most Mapuche live in patrilineal extended families (though it is not always the case that families living in the same communities are kin). Each nuclear family owns a plot of land, which is cultivated for subsistence and some small-scale selling or trade. Most Mapuche people living in rural areas of the Araucanía region have close ties to urban life, particularly Temuco, the regional capital, and Santiago, through relatives, work, and studies.

The Mapuche maintained political and territorial autonomy south of the Biobío river throughout the Spanish colonial administration of what is today Chile (since the sixteenth century until the nineteenth century). After the arrival of the Spanish, the Mapuche became cattle ranchers and developed an extensive network of commerce with the Spanish (and later the Chileans), with whom they traded livestock and textiles for iron, wine, and silver, among other goods. The political and territorial independence of the Mapuche as a people continued for decades after the Chilean War of Independence (1810–1818), and only came to an end through war three or four generations ago (Bengoa 1996, 2002; Cayuqueo 2017).

The current state of the Mapuche in Chile has its origins in the occupation of their territory by the Chilean army, a military campaign started in 1861 and completed in 1883. After the war, surviving Mapuche were displaced to reservations (S: *reducciones*), where they were forced to make a living out of subsistence agriculture. From a territory that covered 10 million hectares and stretched from the Pacific to the Atlantic, the Mapuche were "reduced" to a territory of approximately 500,000 hectares (Bengoa 1996, 2002). As Bengoa (2002: 61) argued, this is the colonial origin of the current poverty and marginality of the Mapuche rural world.

The state of Chile handed over property rights to the defeated Mapuche through a legal instrument called Merced Titles (S: *Títulos de Merced*). The Chilean state handed 3,078 Merced Titles between 1884 and 1919, which corresponded to about 500,000 hectares and benefited 78,000 people (Bengoa 2002: 356). According to Bengoa (ibid.), this was a slow and bureaucratic process that resulted in many Mapuche groups not receiving property rights. Instead, they were forcibly displaced by national and foreign colonists (S: *colonos*) who were eager to appropriate Mapuche lands. Moreover, many Mapuche who did receive property rights subsequently lost their titles due to forced displacement and legal trickery. Bengoa (ibid.: 69) points out that 200 communities with Merced Titles disappeared in the first decades of the twentieth century and, with them, Mapuche lands, which passed into private hands. These lands, which were handed to the Mapuche by the Chilean state and later ended in private hands through illegal means, are being claimed today by Mapuche activists who refer to them as usurped lands (S: *tierras usurpadas*).

Mapuche Studies

There is a vast amount of academic literature on the Mapuche, whose exhaustive review exceeds the scope of this book. Thus, I focus on relatively recent works that have had influence on our current understanding of the Mapuche. Most scholars on the Mapuche would agree on the fundamental contribution of the historian José Bengoa. His work *Historia del pueblo mapuche* (History of the Mapuche People), first published in 1985 and followed by numerous re-editions, inaugurated a new interest in the Mapuche by both scholars and the Chilean public. Bengoa portrays the Mapuche as complex social actors, with internal divisions, struggles and differences, trying to resist or make alliances with both the Spanish and, after the War of Independence (1810–1818), the Chileans. In addition, this historian gave the Mapuche a history of their own vis-à-vis the history of colonial Chile and the Chilean Republic. Remarkably, Bengoa relied on oral narratives (as well as written records) as valid historical sources, giving voice to current Mapuche.

The publication of this foundational academic work was closely followed by Mapuche political mobilization with the advent of democracy in 1990 (this is discussed further later). Moreover, in 2002, Bengoa published a historical essay entitled *Historia de un conflicto. El Estado y los mapuches durante el siglo XX* (History of a Conflict: The State and the Mapuche in the 20th Century). Unlike his 1985 book, aimed primarily at historians and academics, this book is an enjoyable and easy-to-read essay directed at the general public. In this way, in addition to his academic contribution, Bengoa has contributed to the political debate in Chile and his findings as a historian are known beyond the confines of the academy.

Other Chilean historians and social scientists joined the renewed interest in the Mapuche. *Organizaciones, líderes and contiendas Mapuche* (Mapuche Organizations, Leaders, and Contests), by Rolf Foerster and Sonia Montecinos, published in 1988, was also influential in promoting the interest of scholars and the broader public in the Mapuche. The book is a historical and sociological account, based mostly on the review of newspapers, of the varying Mapuche political organizations of the first half of the twentieth century and how they negotiated with the state. In the same vein, Pinto's *La formación del Estado y la nación, y el pueblo Mapuche. De la inclusión a la exclusión* (The Formation of the State and the Nation, and the Mapuche people: From Inclusion to Exclusion) (2003) is an account of how Mapuche were excluded from nation-building discourses and practices in the second half of the nineteenth century, coinciding with the preparations of the military campaigns aimed at conquering Mapuche territory. The exclusion of the Mapuche from the nation, together with military aggression, displacement, and expropriation, as Pinto argued, occurred after a colonial and republican period in which the Mapuche border and autonomy were accepted and conflict was contained through commerce and diplomacy.

Two historians who have published more recently, and in English, are Florencia Mallon and Joanna Crow. Mallon's *Courage Tastes of Blood* (2005) narrates the history of the Mapuche community Nicolas Aillío. The historian also relies on oral narratives to construct the history of a Mapuche community entangled with significant national events, such as the agrarian reform of the 1960s, the repression and brutality of the Pinochet dictatorship (1973–1990), and the recovery of democracy in 1990. Crow's *The Mapuche in Modern Chile: A Cultural History* (2013) focuses on varying cultural productions, such as Mapuche poetry and museums, as well as political discourses from both Mapuche and Chilean leaders, to trace conflicting Mapuche and Chilean discourses regarding Mapuche and national identity. Significantly, this book challenges the common assumption that *indigenismo*, as a political ideology, has been absent from nation-building discourses and practices in Chile.

Another significant event in Mapuche scholarship is the emergence of Mapuche scholars. A collective study group called *Comunidad de historia mapuche* (Mapuche History Community) was founded in 2004 and initially started publishing articles and books online both in Spanish and Mapudungun. The publication of the book *¡... Escucha, wingka ...! Cuatro ensayos de Historia Nacional Mapuche y un epílogo sobre el futuro* (Listen, *wingka*! Four Essays on Mapuche National History and One Epilogue About the Future) (Marimán et al. 2006) by a prestigious national editorial (LOM) made the group well-known among academics and activists. The authors defined their work as a 'cry of the colonized towards other colonized, and at the same time, toward the colonizer, in order to rewrite history to place in it one of the least heard voices' (ibid.: 10, my translation). Another prolific Mapuche journalist, writer and activist is Pedro Cayuqueo, published the book *Historia secreta mapuche* (Secret Mapuche History) (2017). This book is a chronicle about Mapuche history based on the work of historians, anthropologists, and other academics, and, also, on the journalistic report that Cayuqueo made in museums, archives, and libraries in Chile and Argentina. Significantly, this book explores the war against the Mapuche by both the Chilean and Argentinian armies, together with the role of Mapuche political leaders in resisting the invasion. Cayuqueo's intention is to demonstrate that this war, which occurred only three or four generations ago, is the origin of the current political conflict between the Mapuche and the Chilean and Argentinian nation-states. This is in line with Bengoa's (1996, 2002) and Pinto's (2003) work, as detailed previously.

Anthropologists have also contributed to recent accounts of the Mapuche. Regarding Mapuche healing practices, the work of Ana Mariella Bacigalupo is probably one of the most influential. Bacigalupo's *Shamans of the Foye Tree: Gender, Power and Healing Among Chilean Mapuche* (2007), is an ethnographic account of Mapuche shamanism. The book shows how shamanic practices and discourses construct ideas of gender, healing, and race by appropriating, and at the same time transforming and challenging, ideas, values, and aesthetics from Catholicism, the Chilean state and biomedicine. Bacigalupo's more recent publication *Thunder Shaman: Making History with Mapuche Spirits in Chile and Patagonia* (2016) is a collaborative project between the anthropologist and the Machi Francisca Kolipi. In this work, Bacigalupo shows how machi construct history by their embodiment of the past. Machi embody the spirits of deceased shamans, and they ritually perform their ancestors' memories and experiences. In this way, machi embodiment and performance of the past challenge positivistic understandings of history as progress and of time as linear.

The most recent published ethnography on Mapuche healing practices in English is Kristensen's *Patients, Doctors and Healers: Medical Worlds Among the Mapuche of Southern Chile* (2019). This work is a study of Mapuche medicine and medical pluralism in the south of Chile, with a focus on medical narratives by patients. By exploring the motivations behind Indigenous and non-Indigenous people choosing Mapuche medicine, the author postulates that this choice is a way of expressing and transforming a social position of marginality, generating inter-ethnic solidarity bonds among marginal individuals, and expressing discontent with the Chilean public health system and its inherent inequalities.

This ethnography builds on the ones mentioned above in the sense that it considers Mapuche shamanism as a practice embedded in larger political contexts, which should be taken into consideration. In addition, this work seeks to expand on previous scholarship on Mapuche shamanism by focusing on healing techniques and their transformative capacities. In this way, Mapuche ritual healing is understood not only as a political strategy of resistance and subversion, but also as a world and people making practice, which can create the experience of both a collective and a personal Mapuche identity.

The Mapuche Machi

Machi are people with the spiritual gift (S: *don*) to heal and communicate with the spiritual world (Bacigalupo 2007; Cooper 1946; Faron 1997). Machi's abilities derive from a *pülli* (lineage spirit) who communicates with a machi through signs, such as *peuma* (dreams), *perimontun* (visions) and *küymin* (ritual trance). A machi's *pülli* chooses the most suitable member of a family to become a machi. If a machi's *pülli* runs through a particular family, it will continue to endlessly produce new machi among members of the same lineage. A machi's *pülli* is usually (though not exclusively) inherited from the mother's side, after the last member of the family who possessed it dies. This can occur immediately after a machi's death or it can take a long time if a spirit decides there are no suitable candidates in a generation of a family. In addition, some chosen people may refuse to accept the spirit. This refusal usually brings illness and misfortune both to the individual and the whole lineage. Succession, then, does not follow the logic of the firstborn, rather it can skip generations or choose descendants born in any order.

It is a well-known anthropological observation that spiritual healers undergo a long period of illness and misfortune as part of an initiation process. For instance, Lewis (2003: 62–63), following a famous phrase from T.S. Elliot, referred to shamans as a "wounded surgeon," one who overcomes the painful experience of an arduous initiation process and emerges out of it empowered. This is also the case among machi. Usually, a young person, between the age of thirteen to twenty-five, receives a machi call (S: *llamado de machi*) indicating that they have been chosen by their lineage spirit to become a machi. The call occurs in the form of illness and misfortune, and also other signs, such as dreams and visions. What usually occurs is that the machi-to-be becomes very ill without apparent explanation. As is shown in the example that follows (and also in Chapter 4), young people called to be a machi are often sick for years and in a debilitating way. To recover health and wellbeing the person who is being called should accept the call to become a machi and start an initiation process with the help of an experienced machi. The duration of the initiation process varies but it usually lasts several years, including initial perplexity, confusion and reluctance to accept the machi call. Reluctance to become a machi derives from the fact that being a machi is risky, given that machi are constantly exposed to evil spirits, illness and death, and arduous, because it requires constant commitment.

A Mapuche woman, who was a university teacher, narrated the following regarding her sixteen-year-old daughter's machi call and initiation process:

> My eldest son became ill. He was studying to become a teacher at the university. He was throwing his books away, he couldn't study. We took him to see a machi who said the boy was not meant to live in the city because the city is boiling evil [S: *la ciudad es un hervidero de maldad*]. [Instead] he must take care of the *menoko* [wetland], the *mahuiza* [forest], the mountains. That's why he couldn't finish his studies. The machi also told us that in this place a machi is going to be anointed [S:[*se va a levantar una machi*]. In this place, we will know about remedies, there is a machi *pülli* [lineage spirit] fluttering around. The machi did two or three jobs [S: *trabajos*] to my son. In one of those, my daughter went crazy [S: *empezó a rallar la papa*].
>
> After this, my daughter became very ill. She used to tell me: "The teacher speaks but I am not there, I don't want to know anything of what they are teaching me." In that way, she started to hate what is not hers [Western education], to liberate what is her own [Mapuche knowledge]. She could not finish school. During the weekend, she was fine at home in the countryside. We used to send her to school [in the nearest town] and on Tuesday she was not able to go anymore.

> My daughter started saying that a police officer was protecting her. I thought that was a good sign. But a *papai* [respected woman], who stayed at my place, told me that she saw a police officer standing by my daughter's bed all night long. It was the devil. We took her to a private cardiologist who said she had nothing, the tests showed nothing. That helped us make up our minds. We took my daughter to a machi who had to do an exorcism. That was the first job we had to do to my daughter, to take the devil out of her, an exorcism. She resisted violently, she was begging us to take her home, but we had to understand that it was not her but the devil talking …
>
> (Araucanía 2017, interview)

The narration above contains common traits of machi initiation processes. There is an initial sign that a machi will be anointed in a particular place, community or family. In this case, an experienced machi announced it when treating the eldest son of the family. Also, the vignette shows that the young initiate undergoes a period of illness and suffering. Noteworthy is the fact that the family's conviction that the affliction was of a spiritual nature was enhanced by the fact that biomedical testing showed no alterations. The case also shows how a machi should renounce salient social activities, in this case, formal secondary education. To become a machi is a full-time occupation. The fact that the machi's mother, who was a professional who completed higher education, was willing to give up on her daughter completing secondary education is striking. It shows how valuable machi are for families and communities and how committed a family can become in completing the initiation process of a daughter or a son.[2]

Machi divine illnesses and misfortunes and possess the spiritual knowledge to treat them. They deal mostly with spiritual afflictions, but they also treat common ailments to which naturalistic explanations are ascribed. The most common divinatory technique used by machi today is *willentun* or uroscopy (described in Chapter 2). It involves the visual inspection of a patient's bottled urine with the aim of knowing or divining the patient's concerns and troubles. Bacigalupo (2007: 32–33; 60–63) described other divinatory techniques, such as divination through drumming and trance. The most common *lawen* (remedy) prescribed consists of herbal medical infusions, which machi prepare at their private homes. The medicinal herbs used in these preparations are gathered by the machi and their family, received as a gift from friends and patients, and/or bought in local markets and shops.

Machi are the only individuals with the ability to experience *küymin* (ritual trance), which is the ritually induced spirit possession of a machi. While in trance, a machi is possessed by their *pülli* (lineage spirit), who talks through them in the form of a sung prayer and other actions. Ritual trance is usually carried out at the *rewe* (altar), which is a carved tree trunk set in the ground. The *rewe* resembles a pillar-like sacred altar and has an anthropomorphic face at its tip. While in trance, the machi usually climbs to the tip of the *rewe*, performing a machi's ascent to the sky or spiritual world. Therefore, machi are considered bridges or communicators with the spiritual world.

The special ability of machi to deliver a spiritual message transforms them into a vehicle to know the Mapuche past and create Mapuche memory. Because Mapuche *kimün* (ancestral knowledge) has been widely lost due to colonization, it needs to be recovered. There are several ways to recover *kimün* according to my interlocutors: the content of the Mapuche language, which has resisted colonization; the wisdom of the elders, who remember how things used to be; and dreams, which constitute a social relation with ancestors and spirits. Among these varying forms of recovering *kimün*, machi's ability to experience *küymin* (ritual trance) is highly valued. *Küymin* constitutes a direct relation with an ancestor, the spirit of a dead shaman, who can then become lived experience through ritual actions over a machi's body. In this way, machis' ritual actions are indispensable for the creation of a shared Mapuche memory. They are also a Mapuche way of knowing the past through ritual actions in the present.

What a friend told me regarding the initiation ritual of a young male machi is compelling. It shows the recreation of the past in the present so that the past can become a lived experience susceptible to transformation.

> Today there is more stability. We overcame that moment when we were afraid that we [the Mapuche] would disappear. That was seen from above [the sky, heaven] and a couple of years ago many machi began to surface [S: *empezaron a aparecer muchas machi*].
>
> There is a young machi with the spirit of Lautaro [a Mapuche warrior of the sixteenth century]. We think Lautaro was a machi. In a ceremony,

> he [the young machi possessed by Lautaro's spirit] grabbed the *wiño* [a wooden cane used to play ritual hockey or *palin*] and started fighting. Lautaro left here in the middle of the war and now returned fighting! We had to calm him down and explain to him that we were in another era, that we had lost the war. He already understood and is calmer now. Many spirits from the past are coming back and they suffer from seeing us *awingkados* [Westernized].
>
> (Araucanía 2017, interview)

My friend described the ritual performance of a famous Mapuche warrior from the sixteenth century, Lautaro, who was killed by the Spanish *conquistadores* in 1557, returning to the Mapuche world through possessing the body of a young male machi. Stated otherwise, the young initiate was possessed by the spirit of a dead shaman, in this case the famous Mapuche warrior Lautaro. Upon returning, Lautaro realized his people had lost the war and the society he knew no longer existed. He tried to keep fighting but convinced himself that the war was inevitably lost. As mentioned, the ritual in which this occurred was conducted as part of the initiation process of a young male machi. Before the ritual was performed, the young initiate was constantly irritated and enraged. I was told that, after the ritual, the young machi was calmer. So was his spirit, Lautaro, who was becoming reconciled with the new situation of the Mapuche as subjugated to the Chilean state.

There are two important changes that machi have undergone in the twentieth century and that coincided with the Chilean state domination of the Mapuche: machi emerged as predominantly female and as the primary Mapuche religious figure to the detriment of other religious authorities (Degarrod 1998). Nowadays, female machi outnumber male machi by far, to the point where some Chileans think machi are exclusively female. Some Mapuche scholars have emphasized that the feminization of machi in public discourse is related to the colonial association between femininity, witchcraft and Indigenous practices (e.g., Rodríguez and Quidel 2016). There is no consensus on whether the transition to a predominantly female shamanism was from a completely masculine (Cooper 1946) or a mixed gender (Faron 1997) one. There is also no consensus on the historical period in which men were marginalized from shamanism (Degarrod 1998). In her ethnography about Mapuche shamanism and gender, conducted during the 1990s,

Bacigalupo (2007: 164–211) describes how male machi struggle to conform to normative ideas of masculinity through the identification with warriors, doctors and priests.

Until the twentieth century, the *ngillatun* or fertility ritual (described in detail in Chapter 2) was led by male *longko* (headmen) and *ngenpin* (male orators or masters of words). Nowadays, some *ngillatun* rituals are led by male *longko* and *ngenpin* (e.g., Course 2011: 138–59) while others are led by male or female machi (e.g., Bacigalupo 2007: 64–72). Machi presiding over *ngillatun* rituals is a recent occurrence in Mapuche history (ibid.: 70–71). As stated previously, it shows that machi have expanded their area of expertise and authority to the detriment of other religious and political authorities. Some of my interlocutors told me that exclusively male traditional authorities, such as *longko* and *ngenpin*, were perceived as fragile and have lost people's trust.

Also, some male friends commented that it was possible that men had committed many moral and spiritual transgressions in the past, such as betrayals in their negotiations with the Chilean invaders. For this reason, female machi had to take control over *ngillatun* rituals. Bacigalupo (ibid.: 70) described two reasons why her informants thought machi took control over the *ngillatun* ritual: young men were no longer interested in becoming ritual orators, and machi, contrary to male orators, had God's support.

The Current Political Situation of the Mapuche in Chile

Since the beginning of the democratic transition in 1990, Mapuche political activism has focused on the recovery of usurped lands, political autonomy and the recognition of a plurinational state. Mapuche activism has been received ambiguously by the Chilean state. On the one hand, there has been permanent police repression, including illegal prosecution and killing of Mapuche activists. The last tragic killing occurred in 2018 when Camilo Catrillanca was shot dead by the police while he was unarmed and driving his tractor.[3] On the other hand, there have been some attempts to grant cultural rights and recognition to the Mapuche. For instance, Chile's ratification of the International Labour Organization Convention on Indigenous and Tribal Peoples (or ILO-convention 169) (1989) in 2009, the implementation of intercultural education programs and, significantly for this work, the public financing of Mapuche medicine in general primary care centers and exclusive Mapuche medicine centers. In this way, the state is divided between the use of coercive force and the understanding of the Mapuche as the internal enemy and attempts to persuasively delimit and manage cultural difference.

Mapuche political activism since the 1990s coincides with a continental phenomenon that Hale (1994, 1997) has described as the emergence of cultural politics of identity. As this phenomenon has been understood as part of a neoliberal form of governance, it has also been framed as neoliberal multiculturalism (e.g., Hale 2005). Several scholars (e.g., Collier 1994; Gabriel 1994; Hale 1994, 1997, 2005) have pointed out that there has been a historical shift in grassroots movements in the Americas. This has been a shift from the national-popular movements based on class divisions of the 1960s, to the construction of different identities as unique and differentiated and inherently endowed with fundamental rights. In this way, different political minorities such as women, Afro-descendant peoples, LGBT peoples, and Indigenous peoples advance a political discourse based on cultural difference and recognition. Emblematic of this shift was the surge of political activism by Indigenous peoples throughout the Americas on the Columbus Quintecenary in 1992 (Gabriel 1994).

As Hale has pointed out: "we can also note that indigenous peoples now increasingly advance their struggles through a discourse that links Indian identity with rights to territory, autonomy, and peoplehood – rights that run parallel to those of the nation-state itself" (Hale 1997: 571).

On the Columbus Quintecenary in 1992, the Mapuche joined the continental protests and participated in international meetings (Gabriel 1994). The resistance campaign was not only against the old conquest, but also against a new one led by foreign corporativism through the creation of new forms of dependence through trade agreements and extractivism. Since that moment, several Mapuche political organizations have proliferated. Most of these organizations advance a discourse based on the recognition of an Indigenous identity different from that of the rest of the Chilean society (Bengoa and Caniguan 2012). In its more radical expression, there have been some groups advancing the idea of a totally autonomous Mapuche state (though most groups advance the idea of political autonomy within one plurinational state).

Overall, Mapuche political discourse today shows a clear resistance to the idea of racial mixture (S: *mestizaje*) as the source of a unitary national identity (e.g., Cayuqueo 2017). Racial mixture had been at the core of nation-building discourses throughout the twentieth century and consists of the idea that Chilean people are all part of the same mixed race and culture. This mixed race and culture derives from the historical encounter between the Spanish and Indigenous peoples and is the origin of one homogenous nation. In contrast, Mapuche politics of identity consists of establishing a unique identity endowed with fundamental rights. Neoliberal governance has reinforced Mapuche politics of identity (and vice versa) and, thus, it has moved away from racial mixture as a nation-building discourse toward delimiting and managing difference (or toward a multicultural discourse).

The Mapuche resistance against the ideology of racial mixture had its peak of political strength in the election of the Constitutional Convention in 2021. The elected Convention was chaired by a Mapuche woman, Elisa Loncón, and included reserved Indigenous seats. The constitutional proposal issued by the Convention was rejected in 2022 by 62 percent of the Chilean voters. The proposal for Chile to become a plurinational state, made by both the Chilean left and Indigenous representatives, was probably one of the leading reasons Chileans overwhelmingly rejected the constitutional proposal. Thus, we have been witnessing a revival of the idea of racial mixture as a nation-building discourse. Some sectors of the traditional right and the far right continue to defend the idea of racial mixture (S: *mestizaje*) as the historical and racial origin of one Chilean nation. Therefore, they refuse to grant cultural rights to Indigenous groups, such as reserved seats in Congress or Constitutional recognition.

The shift from the idea of racial mixture (S: *mestizaje*) as a nation-building discourse to the idea of cultural identity and rights is a relevant political transformation. It has opened the door to new opportunities for negotiation that, although highly unequal, have allowed the Indigenous movements valuable conquests. In this way, the ideology of cultural difference has extended citizenship to those who were previously excluded from the state. In addition, multiculturalism has also transformed cultural difference into a commodity, through things such as tourism and arts and crafts, and is, thus, a vehicle and a consequence of the neoliberal market expansion (De la Cadena 2015: 163).

However, multicultural politics have been the object of fierce criticism. Viveiros de Castro (e.g., 2004) has famously argued that while multiculturalism is based on a Western distinction between nature and culture, where nature is one and culture is plural; Amazonian cosmologies imagine a world with "spiritual unity and corporeal diversity" (ibid.: 6), which was framed as multinaturalism. In turn, Viveiros de Castro's idea of different ontologies between the West and, in the case at hand, Amazonian cosmologies, has been criticized on the basis of its essentializing nature of both the West and Amazonian cultures. De la Cadena (2010, 2015) has also asserted that multiculturalism is insufficient to understand Indigenous politics in South America today, given the fact that Indigenous movements propose a new understanding of politics that is not only based on the participation of different bodies marked by gender, race, sexuality or ethnicity, but also on the participation of non-human persons, such as a living sacred mountain whose life is threatened by a mining project. The participation of elements of nature as persons or "earth beings" (De la Cadena 2015) in political debates subverts the dichotomy of nature/culture at the heart of multicultural politics. Therefore, De la Cadena (ibid.: 31) stresses the way in which Indigenous politics supposes "an important challenge to the state politics [of] recognition and its incapacity of considering the being of what it does not know." Instead of emphasizing the incommensurability of different ontologies, De la Cadena understands indigeneity in Cuzco as mutually and historically constituted with non-indigeneity. Thus, she conceives of things Indigenous and things non-Indigenous as "partial connections" (ibid.: 32): "intra-related" (instead of inter-related) collectives, which "resist being divided into parts and wholes" (ibid.: 32).

Mapuche medical practices and machi have been fundamental in Mapuche politics regarding territory, autonomy and identity. Already at the international meetings that took place on the Columbus Quintecenary, different Indigenous peoples of the Americas raised the need to gain state recognition for Indigenous medical practices (Gabriel 1994). Medical practices not only provide a unique identity and enact a collective memory but also allow the political participation of non-human actors such as spirits and ancestors. For instance, political discourses against extractivism are not only based on the need to protect local agriculture and tourism but also on the necessity of avoiding spiritual punishment by the *ngen* (spiritual guardians or owners) of rivers and mountains. In this way, extractive projects, such as mining or timber production, are understood as spiritual transgressions and, as such, are a common cause of spiritual illnesses and ailments that should be prevented not only through ritual healing action but also through political activism.

The development and implementation of intercultural health initiatives by the Chilean Ministry of Health has been one of the most important multicultural neoliberal policies. State-led intercultural health initiatives began in Araucanía region in the early 2000s and then expanded to other regions, including Santiago. At the time in which I conducted fieldwork, there were four intercultural medical centers in Araucanía. These intercultural medical facilities were in Imperial, Puerto Saavedra, Boroa and Makewe, and one was being constructed in Galvarino. They are funded through the regional office of the Ministry of Health, and they also receive funding through municipalities. These initiatives are the result of negotiations between Mapuche organizations and health authorities. These negotiations have not occurred without conflict, which has been centered around the degree of autonomy of Mapuche organizations in administering state-funded Mapuche centers (e.g., Vargas 2018). For instance, I attended a meeting in which a machi, who was also a founder member of a Mapuche organization administering a state-funded Mapuche medical center, said the following: "The State should finance, because it is our right, but it should not regulate." Not surprisingly, state authorities disagreed and, instead, postulated that they should regulate what they finance due to issues of accountability.

The Mapuche scholar, Andrés Cuyul (2013, 2015), proposes a critique of multiculturalism in health policies in Chile. He argues that the ideology of "tolerance" in intercultural health policies contributes to making health disparities and unequal power relations invisible. Cuyul (2013) has also argued that machi working in state-funded medical centers bureaucratizes machi practices and, thus, transforms them into "clinical" practices instead of "socio-spiritual" ones. Moreover, Cuyul (ibid.) is concerned with possible health consequences for machi who work in public clinics, given the fact that this is a transgression susceptible to negative spiritual consequences in the Mapuche cosmogony.

Organization of the Chapters

This book is organized as follows. Chapter 1 is a theoretical chapter that seeks to locate this ethnographic account of Mapuche healing transformations in the context of a relevant anthropological problem. I seek to provide a theoretical rationale for healing transformations that can account for the complementarity of embodied and symbolic transformations. In the first part of the chapter, I draw on developments within anthropology (e.g., Csordas 1993; Hsu 2005, 2015; Ots 1994; Ozawa-De Silva 2006), which demonstrate that at least some aspects of healing transformations are non-symbolic. Non-symbolic healing transformations occur in the form of reorganizations of sensory experience, affective states and bodily habits. In the second part of the chapter, I explore how symbolic elaborations are grounded in the body. To do so, I draw on Csordas' (1990, 1994a, 1994b) phenomenological understanding of the self as an indeterminate and relational process that starts in pre-reflexive bodily experience and ends in mental representations. Also, I attend to imagination as a mode of self-process or a mode in which the self moves from indeterminacy to objectification.

Chapter 2 explores ethnographically what my informants explicitly considered made a machi a real machi: to see and treat illnesses and misfortunes effectively and to preside over *ngillatun* rituals (and other community ceremonies) effectively. The chapter is mostly based on ethnographic observations of one machi's practice: a popular and successful healer whom I call Machi Carmen. I also make comparisons to the practice of other machi. The first part of the chapter focuses on the *pewtun* ritual or uroscopy, which is a divinatory technique. *Pewtun* is a ritual in which the machi "sees" the illness or problem in a patient's bottled urine and is, then, able to prescribe *lawen* (remedies) and other solutions. *Pewtun* techniques promote the patient's imaginative engagement with the therapeutic procedure through the manipulation of attention and the emotions. Thus, for a successful *pewtun* to be accomplished, a machi needs to promote the active participation of the patient. In the second part of the chapter, I explore the role of Machi Carmen as the presiding ancestral authority of the *ngillatun* ritual. The effective performance of the *ngillatun* ritual gives an opportunity for the exchange of feelings of belonging and shared self-worth. In this way, Machi Carmen can strengthen her role as a healer and community builder, preventing illnesses and misfortunes through her ability to enter *küymin* (ritual trance) and deliver a message from the spirits to the community.

Chapter 3 continues to explore how machi can see illnesses and misfortunes. Here, I focus on illnesses and ailments caused by *wekufe* (evil spirits). Healing techniques described in this chapter aim at making the evil spirit visible and, thus, exteriorizing it, weakening it and making it vulnerable to ritual healing actions. The preferred sensory modality of "seeing" is vision, but other modalities, such as touch and sound, are also relevant. Machi use different techniques to promote the imaginative seeing of evil spirits, which include the circulation of negative emotions, such as fear, the manipulation of attention and the effect on the senses of different bodily techniques such as massage or chanting. The chapter discusses two ritual events directed against evil spirits. The first one corresponds to a case of witchcraft in which a family, with the help of a machi, searches for a buried object attached to an evil spirit (S: *entierro*) left in their courtyard by a witch. The second case refers to unintended consequences when dealing unsuccessfully with evil spirits. It tells the story of Rosa, a woman who was hospitalized for a diabetic coma and had to be reintegrated into her family life after a long absence. Both cases illustrate the significance of imaginative seeing through varied healing techniques in ritual healing performative efficacy.

Chapter 4 explores doubts and failure in ritual healing to further enrich the understanding of Mapuche ritual healing efficacy. Here, I explore ethnographically events in which doubts are expressed regarding the efficacy of a particular healing action or the authenticity of a healer. I follow ideas on ritual healing failure as a performance failure or imperfection (Grimes 1990; Schieffelin 1996, 2007). I focus on two case studies. The first case relates to a machi, Ana, who had lost the ability to heal because her spirit had abandoned her. To make the spirit return to the machi's body, a *zatun* ritual was performed. The machi's performance was judged by many of the participants as indicative of her inauthenticity as a machi, a concern expressed as doubts regarding whether Ana was, in fact, a real machi. These doubts originated in a series of mishaps among which the most significant one was the deployment of inappropriate emotions while in trance (i.e., the machi cried while in trance). The second case study describes the difficulties of a *machil* (machi initiate), Marta, in satisfactorily completing her initiation process. Unlike the case above, Marta's difficulties in becoming a machi were not explained by an imperfect performance, but by her reluctance to perform. In turn, her resistance to perform derived from what she perceived as a lack of spiritual inspiration or her inability to understand the spirits' messages.

Finally, Chapter 5 links ritual healing bodily transformations with Mapuche politics of identity. Specifically, this chapter seeks to link ethnographically embodied and discursive practices regarding the *wetripantü* ritual or the "Mapuche New Year" and its interaction with Mapuche struggles for identity, memory and authenticity. Here, I follow Csordas' (1999) methodological proposition of examining the links between ritual healing and identity politics at a political, social and individual level. At a political level, *wetripantü* celebrations discursively create a Mapuche identity that is unique and, thus, different to the rest of Chilean society. The fundamental Mapuche claim is that to celebrate the New Year in December is "scientifically" wrong in the Southern Hemisphere, a claim derived from Mapuche ancestral understanding of nature. At a social level, *wetripantü* celebrations allow for negotiations between conflicting Mapuche identities, such as gender and religious identity. In this way, ritual practice not only enhances difference from the rest of society, but it also articulates difference and conflict within Mapuche society. Lastly, I describe the perspective of a Mapuche man who participated in a *wetripantü* celebration. At an individual level, ritual engagement facilitates making sense of various individual difficulties in relation to a shared Mapuche identity, which is a source of dignity and self-worth. In this way, ritual healing does not only have an existential function but also a political one, which is manifested through the ways in which Mapuche actors attempt to control Mapuche identity at a political, social, and individual level.

In conclusion, this ethnography examines Mapuche healing efficacy through a phenomenological perspective, with careful attention to the social and political context. The aim is to understand how a machi can see an illness or problem and prescribe remedies and solutions that can be perceived as efficacious. Thus, the focus of this work is on healing techniques that can allow machi to see an illness or a problem and transform a problematic situation. In addition, this work explores the significance of Mapuche medical practices in collective struggles for memory, identity and wellbeing.

Notes

1. All names are pseudonyms.
2. The son's illness narrated at the beginning of this extract was also interpreted as a spiritual call. In his case, the call was to become a *longko* (headman), which is also considered a spiritual gift as described in Chapter 4. While my friend's daughter had to abandon secondary education, her son dropped out of university.
3. This case prompted massive nationwide street protests in an unprecedented display of solidarity by the Chilean public toward the Mapuche of the south. It was hugely covered by the Chilean press (see, for example, Basadre 2018) and it also received attention by the international press (see Bartlett 2018). In addition, the image of Camilo Catrillanca, together with the Mapuche flag, became omnipresent in the street protests and nationwide uprising of October 2019.

Chapter 1
Ritual Transformations of the Self

The purpose of this theoretical discussion is to provide a rationale for positive experiential transformations (or lack of them) in the context of ritual healing. In other words, my interest is in understanding how a person comes to feel better through healing action. The account I give here is one from the perspective of the phenomenology of the body/subject. My argument is divided into two parts. First, I argue that at least some aspects of healing transformations arise from changes in bodily and affective experience that are not mediated by reconfigurations of symbolic meaning. People can experience positive changes while having gained little new discursive meaning about a problem or situation. However, new discursive meaning about a problem or situation can lead to creative ways of dealing with adverse circumstances. It is undeniable that the identification of a problem and the analysis of alternative solutions is extremely important in the therapeutic context. How can we reconcile the observation that the acquisition of new discursive meaning is neither necessary nor sufficient to explain the success of a healing episode or process, but occurs with high frequency in most therapeutic practices? Therefore, the argument stated above, that of healing transformations not always being mediated by reconfigurations of symbolic meaning, needs to be enriched. Mental processes, such as analogy, theory-making and perspective-taking are effective forms of signifying a situation that can solve problems and have therapeutic relevance. Healing involves both narratives that reflexively elaborate experience and pre-reflexive bodily and affective experience. Thus, I intend to explore the mutual relations between bodily and affective pre-reflexive experience and reflexive reconfigurations of symbolic meaning. In this way, the second part of my argument is that a first layer of embodied transformations is necessary for later rearrangements of symbolic meaning. In this way, I intend to link bodily transformations to cultural meanings and constraints. Crossley (1996) wrote that two main theoretical approaches to the body have predominated within social sciences. The body/power is the body historically "inscribed" from the outside, while the body/subject is the phenomenological "lived body." Crossley argued that these two approaches are not incompatible because both are grounded in a conception of the body as historically and socially constituted (as opposed to biologically determined). Within sociocultural anthropology, a transition occurred from an understanding of the body as determined by biology and thus precultural, to symbolic approaches to the body (Asad 1997). Symbolic approaches (e.g., Douglas 1966, 1970) consider the body as a natural symbol of social relations. Following a symbolic approach, anthropologists studying ritual healing (e.g., Frank 1963; Levi-Strauss 1963; Turner 1967) thought that healing transformations occurred as a function of reconfigurations of symbolic meaning and the conventional belief in the power of the healer/shaman.

Symbolic theories have also been influential within the medical sciences, especially within those opposed to biological reductionism (e.g., Kleinman 1980, 1988). Evidence of a placebo effect, present in almost any kind of biomedical procedure, has led to the idea that, in addition to a biological effect, some aspects of medical efficacy are related to the subjective and interpersonal domains of the medical encounter. Moerman (2002) proposed that we understand the placebo effect as the "meaning response," which is "the psychological and physiological effect of *meaning* in the treatment of illness" (ibid.: 14, emphasis in original). In a similar dualistic framework, Kleinman (1973) conceptualized medicine as having a dual reality: "scientific and ordinary," "biophysical and human." This dualistic framework is evident in the belief that to achieve efficacy doctors should be technically competent (which is associated with having a knowledge of basic sciences) but also caring (which is reflected in qualities such as compassion and empathy) (Good and DelVecchio-Good 1993). Kleinman's proposal was to use symbols, especially language, as a way of reconciling social events and psychophysiological responses to them. The idea of the privileged situation of language and verbal communication as a path between dualities explains some medical anthropologists' focus on illness narratives (e.g., Good 1994; Kleinman 1988) to access individual experience in an increasingly protocolized medical culture.

Some anthropological work on ritual healing (e.g., Csordas 1990, 1993, 1994a; Hsu 2005, 2015; Itzhak 2015; Ots 1994) has reached a significant insight, which is the starting point of this theoretical discussion: the realization that we do not know the world, ourselves, and others only through symbolic representations analyzed by a Cartesian mind. When applied to ritual action, the insight mentioned above leads to a different understanding of the efficacy of ritual healing: healing action transforms the body. Thus, meaning does not only arise from the relationship between abstract concepts. Rather, meaning also arises from the connection between abstract concepts and the body/subject with its skills and practices (Kirmayer 1992: 334). Moreover, the body/subject is not only representing something other than itself. Rather, the body/subject has agency and is constitutive of itself and its relationships with others and the world (Csordas 1994b). Throughout this thesis, this anthropological insight will guide my ethnographic exploration of Mapuche medical practices and their potentiality for generating experiential transformations. In doing so, I intend both to contribute to the theoretical problem of medical efficacy from the perspective of the phenomenology of the body/subject, and to conduct an ethnographic exploration of Mapuche ritual transformations grounded in the phenomenology of the body/subject.

My argument does not try to compete with a symbolic approach in explaining therapeutic efficacy. Rather, it complements a symbolic understanding of healing transformations by grounding symbols in the body. I think it is necessary to complement the understanding of healing transformations as being purely symbolic for, at least, the following reasons. First, a consequence of the symbolic understanding of healing transformations is the tendency to elaborate theories of efficacy that share a common understanding of how efficacy is achieved by a limited and unspecific repertoire of global mental mechanisms (Csordas 1994a: 3). These mechanisms include trance, catharsis, placebo effect, and suggestion. But these hypotheses do not offer an explanation as to why and how these mechanisms are effective, if indeed they are. Also, they do not account for cultural specificity, and they tend to be used in pejorative ways. Second, to postulate that a healing effect or change is purely symbolic can lead to the conclusion that it only changes abstract concepts in the mind. Then, little attention is given to healing techniques, skills, and practices and how they transform the body. Contrarily, anthropological evidence on ritual healing shows that different therapeutic techniques, at different historical moments and geographic locations, have developed sophisticated strategies to induce transformation in the human body. Acupuncture, bloodletting, surgery, massage, use of purgatives, hallucinogens, or stimulants are only a handful of well-known examples. Therefore, we must account for the effects in the bodies of people who are undergoing healing experiences. Lastly, symbolic approaches focus on symbols and then try to trace back the relationship between symbols, subjects, and their world. Instead, an approach from the phenomenology of the body/subject focuses on cultural processes that produce both symbols and non-symbolic meaningful experience. Focusing on processes of constitution rather than on already definite endings can allow us to better grasp experiences of transformation and the creation of new meaning.

Here, I understand symbols as a function of textuality and, thus, always primarily related to other symbols and not to subjects and their motives. Thus, a symbol is able to make sense through its relationship with other symbols and it can be progressively (through speech, writing, and printing) expanded and abstracted from the body (Berger 1987). In addition, symbols, as a function of textuality, relate to their objects through convention. However, as I show below, symbols can be taken up into experience through imagination as embodied images. In turn, embodied images can be abstracted from the body and analyzed as a symbol (Csordas 1994a: 74–87). In this way, I draw on Csordas' work on imagination to portray how a semiotic and a phenomenological approach can be complementary and mutually informative.

Non-symbolic Healing Transformations

Sensory and Affective Transformations as the Locus of Healing Action

I will now go back to the first part of my argument. I stated above that the locus of healing action is not only the rearrangement of symbolic meaning such as the reconfiguration of memories and one's life history, the new understanding of a problem, the identification of a cause, or the elaboration of possible solutions. Rather, healing involves bodily and affective changes that are non-symbolic. These bodily and affective changes occur independently of symbolic representation and are experienced as sudden and involuntary. To explore this type of healing transformation I will turn to the insights developed by anthropologists studying sensory experience in the context of ritual in non-Western societies and ritual healing in Western and non-Western societies.[1]

Lewis (1980: 19–20) reached a significant insight in his study of ritual practices among the Gnau of New Guinea: the meaning of ritual is usually obscure even to the people who participate in it. What is explicit about ritual is how to do it but not its meaning. However, for an observer, one clear characteristic of ritual is that it alerts the senses and directs attention to ritual action. It is this characteristic of ritual, its sensory engagement, that promotes an intuitive, immediate relation with ritual action. Thus, an individual's engagement with ritual cannot be explained as a process of reasoning about the rationality of ritual action. Lewis put it this way:

> Elements that are often to be observed in ritual—the aesthetic side of colour, noise and smell; the decorations, singing, the aromatic plants, the formality, stiffness or strangeness of gesture; and the tension translated by a great volume of excited chatter or by a constrained silence … these are all elements which alert the attention and make ritual peculiar, saying "look and listen," not simply "see and hear."
>
> (Lewis 1980: 20)

In this way, Lewis brings our attention to the various and sophisticated forms in which ritual action generates culturally patterned sensory experience and its significance in people's willingness to participate in ritual action. But in which way could the sensory experience induced by ritual action be conducive to ritual transformations? Kapferer (2004) offered an answer to this question when he postulated that the dynamics of a ritual are a property of its performance structure, and that sensory and affective transformations occur within a ritual performance and not outside of it. Thus, the internal dynamics of ritual reorganize sensory and affective experience producing experiential changes in people's bodies. In this way, ritual is not a coded symbolic formation whose interpretation can be reduced to the sociopolitical or psychological aspects of the world outside it. Kapferer concentrates on what he calls the "virtuality of ritual." "Virtuality" does not mean that ritual is a fake reality: rather, it implies that ritual involves the creation of an "imaginal space," where people can reorient themselves to others and their circumstances, and a "technical space," distant from the everyday routine, in which people can actively transform the structures of reality.

So far, I have stated that ritual is a type of performance that reorganizes sensory and affective experience. I will now turn to ritual action that is explicitly carried out with the intention to heal. Csordas (1993) described how ritual healing induces specific somatic experiences that are socially shared (usually between healer and sufferer) and culturally patterned. Csordas called these somatic shared experiences "somatic modes of attention." "Somatic modes of attention" are culturally patterned somatic experiences engaging the body/subject with its surroundings and others. These experiences are spontaneous, which is to say that they occur independently of mental elaborations. Importantly, these experiences are usually shared between people participating in a healing episode or process. In the context of healing, "somatic modes of attention" are deliberately induced to direct attention and promote openness to a reorganization of dispositions, relationships and practices.

In this way, ritual action induces bodily transformations that are social; that is, they involve changes in the relationships between the people who perform different roles in ritual action. Following this line of thought, Hsu (2005) noted that many healing traditions involve a moment in which pain is intentionally inflicted during treatment. Hsu aimed to understand the significance of the moment at which pain is inflicted in therapeutics. In different societies, pain has been intentionally inflicted with the aim of healing. Acupuncture, moxibustion, and pain during initiation rites are illustrative examples. Thus, pain not only has a survival function, but when it is inflicted on a patient, with a demarcated beginning and end, it can awaken and open the patient's body to the environment. Also, as it is accessed immediately through shared somatic and affective experience, pain can create a sense of connectedness and trans-individuality (Seremetakis 1998: 151) that could be experienced as therapeutic.

During an acupuncture session, the moment of needle insertion generates great mutual attention and tension between patient and acupuncturist. "This is the moment of acute pain infliction: often synchronically the patient shivers slightly or catches a breath of air and the doctor sighs with relief or sometimes grunts with satisfaction" (Hsu 2005: 78). It should be emphasized here that the "acute pain" event is a somatic social event, involving at least two people in the case described. Hsu is emphasizing the therapeutic potentialities of the existential continuity of experience at the level of sensory experience. Hsu calls the moment of acute pain infliction a moment of synchronicity, a moment in which everybody involved is grasped by the same sensory event leading to an enhanced connectedness. "In the moment of an acute pain event it is as though the boundaries between the I and the you are broken down, for both you and I are completely overwhelmed by the pain event" (ibid.: 85). Both social bonding and belonging are enhanced here. The focus on the sociality of the senses allows us to disentangle how healing practices are intentionally designed to enhance such trans-individual connectivity. In the therapeutic context, synchronicity refers to techniques by which trans-individual sensory engagement is achieved. The acute pain event can thus be viewed as a trigger for an embodied experience of sociality.

The acute pain event could also refer to the ritual intensification of negative emotions such as sadness. Seremetakis (1998) describes how pain enacted in a mourning ritual in rural Greece mobilizes affect, meanings and values through the community. The mourning ceremony begins with the women's mourning ritual in which women improvise an extended lament. There is one woman, the leading *koriféa*, who is showing the highest intensity of pain and her performance is the center around which other performances are organized. The responses to the leading *koriféa* validate her pain. The acoustic interplay between the leading *koriféa* and the chorus is accompanied by a variety of gestures that also attempt to intensify emotional pain and suffering. The ritual is highly gendered. Women are vocal and demonstrative, while men are silent. Also, men are separated from women. But men are not ignored, they function as a silent chorus. The ritual intensification of emotional pain generates synchronicity, to use Hsu's term, which leads to feelings of connectedness and belonging.

Besides inducing moments of trans-individual connectedness, the technical induction of synchronicity can also open up the person and the group to new dispositions to experience. Thus, the techniques of generating synchronicity induce liminality and the possibility for transformation. As Lewis wrote, ritual action is an invitation to look and listen, a suggestion that something important is going to happen. In this way, the direction of attention through synchronicity promotes imagination and creative ways of dealing with a situation. Thus, healing enhances creativity, understood as the utilization of new meanings and new practices in dealing with everyday reality. The following ethnographic example is illustrative.

To summarize what has been said, moments of synchronicity can be therapeutic in at least two ways. First, they enhance both a sense of belonging and trans-individual connection. Second, since they alert the senses and promote awareness and volition, they predispose a person to new dispositions or reorganizations of experience (Csordas 1993; Desjarlais 1996; Devisch 1990; Hsu 2005, 2015; Seremetakis 1998).

Bodily Habits and Ritual Healing

The way therapeutic techniques modify the body generate non-symbolic meaning. No mental or deliberative cognitive processes are necessary to induce moral states through the manipulation of bodily habits. Here, I explore anthropological work on bodily habits and its relation to morality and identity. This further supports my argument that at least some aspects of healing transformations are non-symbolic.

For Merleau-Ponty (2012: 144) our bodies sediment the past through motor habits or skills (e.g., driving a car or playing the piano). Motor habits are not only about mechanistic repetition, rather they can provide an intentional response to specific situations. Memory, in the form of motor habits, is not a coded motor or emotional response in our brains. Rather, motor habits refer to concrete bodily interactions that are part of our repertoire of body practices. These body practices are acquired pre-reflexively through experience and cultural practices and are susceptible to change and rearrangement. Thus, our body has knowledge and can gain new knowledge through experience. In our everyday routine we engage with our repertoire of body habits by anticipating objects and engaging with them. Again, this is not a mechanistic reaction of the body, but an active encounter with the environment. In other words, pre-reflexive action is not a response to a given stimulus in the external world. Alternatively, the objects, the world, and the other, are encountered through the meeting of our intentionality and the objects in the world to which it is oriented (Merleau-Ponty 2012: 77).

Bourdieu's habitus is significant to continue this discussion given the fact that it locates a body with a past and habits in a cultural world. It provides the body with a cultural history. Thus, the habitus is "an endless capacity to engender products—thoughts, perceptions, expressions, actions—whose limits are set by the historically and socially situated conditions of its production" (Bourdieu 1977: 95).

The habitus is a set of historical relationships incorporated within individual bodies. However, although the habitus can be considered subjective (not just externally imposed or inscribed in the individual), it is not individual, but social. It is a principle that organizes internalized structures, perception, and action common to all members of a social field. It is transmitted through practice without reaching the level of reflexive discourse. It allows the creation of a common-sense world within a group and is also the way each becomes inseparable from the whole and from its history. Bodily habits are inevitably linked to the history of a group—they are "history turned into nature" (Bourdieu 1977: 78).

The habitus is also a way of generating boundaries between different social groups. Thus, the habitus is mediated by taste: "an incorporated principle of classification which governs all forms of incorporation, choosing and modifying everything that the body ingests and digests and assimilates, physiologically and psychologically" (Bourdieu 1986: 190). Taste, then, refers to a principle of establishing identity and boundaries, but also to the sense of taste, being the capacity of differentiating between, and preferring, different foods and flavors.

Bodily habits are means of generating specific affective and moral states. These states can later promote reflexive re-conceptualizations of autobiographical memory and symbolic content within therapeutic contexts. The understanding of healing action as promoting a reconstitution of past memories, so a person can have a new understanding of their past, is a common way of understanding ritual healing efficacy (e.g., Lindquist 2005). In this way, the understanding of the past as sedimented in bodily habits opens up new understandings about how the past can be transformed in the present, not just by the rearrangements of abstract memories in the mind, but by the engagement of the body with a present situation.

Re-conceptualizations of symbolic meaning, including mental elaborations of one's biographical memory, occur in a layer of experience that is reflexive and personal. However, the point I am trying to make is that these interpretations of recollected past events can only be transformed into vivid present experiences through the involvement of the senses, the imagination, and corresponding affective states. Therefore, interpretations about the past can only become vivid experience in the present if the body is performatively involved. Transformations occur in the fitting together of habitual bodily practices and culturally patterned sensorial modalities, with cultural meaning and moral values.

Symbolic meaning, such as autobiographical memory, is, then, generated in social interaction. This does not only mean that it is negotiated through verbal interchanges, but that it emerges from a shared habitus. In this way, individual suffering can arise from the way the body/subject is oriented toward a historical and social milieu (e.g., Pandolfi 2007).

So far, I have indicated that a significant locus of healing ritual action corresponds to affective and sensory experience that is not mediated by reflexive reconfigurations of symbolic meaning. Healing action at this level may be therapeutic in three different ways. First, affective and sensory transformations may promote experiences of trans-individual connection and enhanced belonging and connectedness. Secondly, transformations in sensory and affective experience can predispose the active and creative engagement with a situation, thus promoting volition and action. Lastly, I stated that bodily habits contain moral and cultural meanings. In this way, the manipulation of bodily habits through different bodily techniques can induce certain types of moral and affective dispositions that may lead to constructing new meaning about a problem or situation. The reflective understanding of a problem or situation, then, inevitably starts in the body and its habits, practices, and skills.

Mutual Relations Between Symbolic and Non-Symbolic Healing Transformations

As I stated at the beginning of this discussion, reflexive understandings of a problem or situation play a significant role in therapeutic settings. So far, I have only discussed pre-reflexive transformations in sensory experience, affectivity, and bodily habits as the locus of efficacy. Therefore, in the second part of the chapter I intend to provide a rationale of the mutual relations between symbolic and non-symbolic healing transformations. To do so I draw on the work of Thomas Csordas (1990, 1993, 1994a, 1994b) on ritual transformations among Catholic Charismatics in the U.S. Csordas' work provides a rationale to understand ritual healing's efficacy in culturally specific ways. In doing so, Csordas posits the locus of efficacy in the self (Csordas 1994a). Csordas understands the self as a process that starts in pre-reflexive bodily and affective experience and ends in symbolic representations (including the representation of oneself as a person with a unique set of characteristics). In positing the self as the locus of efficacy, Csordas develops a theory of healing efficacy that relates bodily pre-reflexive experience with reflexive reconfigurations of symbolic meaning. Drawing on Csordas, I argue that a first layer of sudden bodily transformations is necessary to induce reconfigurations of symbols in an experientially meaningful way.

In Csordas' work, imagination is the vehicle through which embodied experience and mental processes are reconciled. Imagination acts as a vehicle that fits together pre-reflexive bodily experience, cultural objects of the milieu, and situated cultural practices. Csordas' theoretical work proposes to complement Pierce's semiotic with Sartre's phenomenological understanding of imagination (Csordas 1994a). Thus, it is possible to complement a semiotic view of healing efficacy as the transformation of symbolic relations, with a phenomenological understanding of efficacy as a rearrangement of pre-reflexive dispositions to the world.

The Cultural Phenomenological Self

What is striking so far in scholarship is that the self has been present in anthropological discussions about diagnosis and etiology, but relatively absent in discussions of the efficacy problem. Going back to Csordas' attempt to posit the self as the locus of efficacy, it becomes evident that there is a need for a theory of the self. Csordas recognizes the existence of the self in culture and language; but he is saying that the self is not an already constituted substance or entity. Rather, it is an open-ended process of self-objectification. Therefore, the self could be better referred to as "self-processes." With ritual healing as the object of his inquiry, Csordas (1990, 1993, 1994a, 1994b) postulates that the individuation of the self and illness is a consequence of dualistic thinking in Western disciplines. Using a phenomenological approach, he proposes to focus on the cultural processes through which the self is objectified, instead of focusing on the already objectified self. The understanding of the self as a constitutive process occurring every time the subject relates with someone is significant to therapeutics. The self, understood in this way, is susceptible to transformations through treatment. However, self-processes occur under cultural and historical constraints. They do not happen in a vacuum. To explain these constraints, Csordas (1990, 1994a) turns to Bourdieu's concept of the habitus. Therefore, in attempting the intellectual and empirical task of defining the self, Csordas follows theoretical developments by Merleau-Ponty (2012) and Bourdieu (1977) in saying that the self is socially situated, prior to any reflexive individuation.

Merleau-Ponty's concept of the pre-objective (Csordas 1990) is key to understanding Csordas' conception of the self. The pre-objective is a concept used by Merleau-Ponty as a way of collapsing the subject-object dualism at the level of perception. In using this concept, Merleau-Ponty goes against the positivist idea that objects in the world have inherent qualities and that perception is a mechanistic process involving the de-codification of sensorial stimulus to nerve impulses by sensorial organs, and the later new de-codification of nerve transmission into motor action, emotion, and meaning in the brain. As an alternative to this idea, Merleau-Ponty posits that perception is a process of objects being constituted through the engagement of the body with the world. There are no objects prior to perception: rather, objects are constituted through perception. In other words, objects do not have inherent qualities—they come to be when the body engages with them. Perception, then, is a process that ends in objects, which are a secondary product of reflexive thinking. However, at the level of perception we are simply "being in the world." To start from the abstraction (or to start for the relation between abstract concepts as in structuralism) and analytically work backward to the perceiving subject does not capture perception as a constitutive process. The pre-objective of being in the world should therefore be the starting point for anthropological empirical research. This idea was framed by Csordas as "embodiment," constituting a proposal of a methodological orientation for ethnographers. Note that the phenomenological body becomes the locus of the self instead of the mind. In this way, the mind becomes the locus of self-objectification (Csordas 1994b), while the locus of subjectivity and agency is the body.

Csordas' approach has been criticized for creating a new subject/object dichotomy (or mind/body dichotomy), when he emphasizes that perception begins in pre-reflexive bodily experience and ends in objects (or mental representations), or when he proposes that the mind is the locus of objectification. For example, Voss (2011) points out that this approach results in a failed attempt to overcome the subject/object duality, while highlighting that "subject and object and thus ownness and foreignness emerge through an incessant process of simultaneous inclusion and exclusion" (ibid.: 171). Nevertheless, in my reading, what Csordas is proposing does not contradict Voss' ideas. According to Csordas (1994a), self and other (and mind and body) are distinctions that arise in self-processes and, thus, are aspects of the same structure: the body/subject (as opposed to two different substances in Cartesian mind/body dualism). However, there is a layer of pre-reflexive experience in which these distinctions blur. The other (including the experience of oneself as other, and the experience of oneself as different to other) is achieved through reflexivity in ongoing processes of individuation. This is in line with Merleau-Ponty's (2012) idea that we never completely finish the process of individuation. Thus, the individualized and objectified self is always in the making, an open-ended process.

In my reading, the reason why Csordas insists on these distinctions (mind/body and subject/object) has to do with their relevance to everyday experience: we can have the experience of being a body and having a body. Thus, overcoming Cartesian dualism is not a matter of abandoning these distinctions as if they did not exist in everyday experience, neither to mix them, nor to reduce one to the other. Rather, the goal of Csordas' concept of self-processes is to attend to processes in which these distinctions appear, so that, for instance, mental processes (understood as the capacity to take the self and others as objects) can be understood in continuity and built upon embodiment, while retaining their specificity.

Nevertheless, the relative predominance of the term "body" over the term "mind" in Csordas' work may be problematic. Ingold (2000) has brought to our attention the problem of emphasizing the term "body" to the exclusion of the term "mind." "Body and mind, after all, are not two separate things but two ways of describing the same thing – or better, the same process – namely the environmentally situated activity of the human organism/person" (ibid.: 171). If phenomenology's intention is to account for reciprocal influences between the bodily pre-reflexive and the minded reflexive in self-processes, we might talk about enmindment as well as embodiment (ibid.: 170). Here I prefer to use the term "pre-reflexive" to describe somatic and affective experience, and reflexive to describe mental elaborations. Again, these terms are not incommensurables, but aspects of the same self-processes. In addition, instead of speaking of mind and body, or subject and object, it is probably clearer to speak about self-processes in which the previous distinctions arise. However, there is a layer of human existence in which these distinctions blur and in which self-processes start.

Why is Bourdieu's habitus relevant to Csordas? The habitus (Bourdieu 1977) is a pre-reflexive system of dispositions that unifies practices and generates them according to conditions in the social world. Csordas seeks to emphasize that the perceptual origin of shared social objects must occur in a historically and socially informed body. This does not happen in a vacuum. It depends on culturally patterned practices and on the particular conditions of the social and political world. The habitus helps to link perceptual processes to cultural constraints and meaning. Thus, a social practice is neither a mechanical reaction determined by past conditions, nor a completely novel phenomenon. Csordas explains the importance of Bourdieu's habitus in his theory of self in the following way: "To conjoin Bourdieu's understanding of the 'habitus' as an unself-conscious orchestration of practices with Merleau-Ponty's notion of the 'pre-objective' suggests that embodiment need not be restricted to the personal or dyadic microanalysis customarily associated with phenomenology, but is relevant as well to social collectivities" (Csordas 1993: 137).

However, the way social practices and institutions shape embodied action and subjectivity is underdeveloped in Csordas' work.

Although there is an explicit recognition of the historicity of the habitual body (and of the ways in which embodied action is constricted by social structure), little attention is paid to the long-term historical processes of change and creation of new cultural meanings. In the same vein, there is little discussion of how the learning of skills and techniques has a political function or a power/control function (as discussed by Foucault (e.g., 1980: 55–63)). Therefore, Csordas' phenomenological approach to the self, and his proposition that self-processes need not be restricted to psychological processes but can also be applied to social processes needs to be complemented by the historical analyses of long-term historical processes and change, and by careful attention to layered power correlations.

Returning to Csordas' discussion of the self, he conceptualizes the self as "an *indeterminate* capacity to engage or become *oriented* in the world, characterized by *effort* and *reflexivity*" (Csordas 1994a: 6, my emphasis). Indeterminate refers to the idea of the self as an open-ended process, always constituting itself. The self is, then, an endless potentiality of becoming a self. This differs from the notion of the self as an already constituted substance or entity. In this way, a phenomenological understanding of self focuses our attention on indeterminate processes of becoming, rather than already constituted objects. Orientation reflects how the self is always in relation to something: it comes to be in its relationship with the world, from which it is inseparable (the world also contains other selves). Effort and reflexivity are characteristics of the self through which self-awareness occurs (ibid.: 14). Effort refers to intentionality and motivation—the effort of abandoning indeterminacy to find orientation. Reflexivity is our capacity of self-objectification and self-awareness, as well as our capacity of objectifying others—thus, our capacity of making culture and creating a social world. This capacity of self-objectification occurs in the fitting together of pre-reflexive bodily experiences and cultural objects of the milieu through structured cultural practices. As Csordas puts it: "[The] self occurs as a conjunction of pre-reflective bodily experience, culturally constituted world or milieu, and situational specificity or habitus. Self-processes are orientational processes in which aspects of the world are thematized, with the result that the self is objectified, most often as a person with a cultural identity or set of identities" (Csordas 1994a: 6).

To clarify Csordas' ideas I will discuss an ethnographic description of deliverance (Csordas 1990), a form of healing among Charismatic Catholics in the U.S. Through deliverance, demons are commanded to leave the body of an afflicted person. Demons that can possess individuals are named after negative emotions, such as guilt or anger, or morally deviant conduct usually related to sexuality. When spirits are commanded to depart from their host they produce a physical manifestation, as a sign of their departure. These manifestations are multiple, like twisting the neck, vomiting, or coughing. In one case study, a reverend commanded, in the name of Jesus, the spirits of masturbation and sexual aberration to leave their hostages' bodies. After the reverend commanded this, a male participant felt that his arms stretched upwards, further than he could naturally reach. After that he felt an electric feeling in his body and at a certain point his hands dropped. As this was happening in a collective healing session, the behavior of spontaneously elevating and then dropping the arms could be observed in several participants simultaneously.

As cultural objects within the cultural milieu, demons have functions that are related to the motivations of the self. Demons are a mirror image of the ideal self and also intelligent beings that can affect one's behavior. Pre-reflexive bodily experiences, such as the sensation of one's arms being elevated involuntarily, are fitted together with cultural objects of the milieu. From this fitting of intentions with cultural objects of the milieu, meaningful experience arises. For Csordas, the pre-objective aspect of the event that is narrated is that the manifestations of the demons are experienced as spontaneous (involuntary). These are original acts of communication that take limited forms because they emerge from people with a shared habitus, which could explain the fact that the experience described is a collective one. There is an immediate, intuitive understanding of the collective gesture of hands being pulled up ("hands off!") as stopping masturbation and of the mild electric feeling following it as the power of God being felt in one's body. The expressive moment that made this form of self-objectification into a healing process was the sense that the person was being released from the demon. The problem is a sense of loss of control to demonic influence, and healing is a release from bondage and a surrender to the will of God. This is different to common interpretations of demonic possession as being a transgression of body boundaries that are related to the conventionally expressed invasive action of the demon, but not to the pre-objective state of the afflicted. Csordas describes two loci at which the pre-objective perception of demons is indeterminate: control (at which point an emotion like anger becomes the demon anger) and generalization (how many demons may emerge).

From the example described above it follows that at least aspects of efficacy rely on shifts of orientation in self-processes. In other words, efficacy relies on pre-reflexive bodily changes that direct attention toward specific objects of the milieu. This is to say that efficacy relies on pre-reflexive or pre-symbolic processes, which are bodily and affective. The mode in which these processes occur is specific to different cultural contexts and different therapeutic techniques. Therapeutic techniques can modulate orientation toward the world through the manipulation of attention, sensory experience, and affective states. In this way, therapeutic techniques manipulating the body generate meaningful experience through exerting bodily transformations. Thus, phenomenologically, meaning is not only a rearrangement, substitution, or introduction of new representations, rather it is a "modulation of being in the world" (Csordas 1994a: 71). In this way, meaning is not always symbolic meaning, rather it can constitute changes in dispositions that are pre-symbolic and can serve as the experiential basis for later symbolic rearrangements of meaning.

Imagination as a Mode of Self-process

How do healing transformations occur through self-processes? To give such an account Csordas turns to imagination phenomenologically understood as a mode of orientation toward the world (Csordas 1994a: 74). Stated otherwise, imagination is a human capacity through which self-processes move from indeterminacy to orientation, from the pre-reflective to reflexive understanding and objectification. Thus, through imagination the subject can engage with the world and others in meaningful ways. Drawing on Casey, Csordas proposes that imagination is embodied, immediate and autonomous (relatively independent from other mental functions such as memory and from context) (Csordas 1994a: 81–84). Csordas describes the spontaneity of imagination in the following way: "it appears suddenly (in a manner that can surprise us), instantaneously (with no time lapse between our intention to produce it and its appearance), and effortlessly (it appears to unfold on its own initiative)" (ibid.: 94). In this way, imagination, as a mode of self-process, acts in the domain of the pre-reflective. Imagination, then, is a mode of orientation. At the same time, imagination is the capacity of reflectively engaging with the world. Thus, imagination is also a mode of self-awareness and self-objectification. Thus, through imagination self-processes can occur starting in bodily sensory experiences and ending in understanding.

Csordas is drawing on a phenomenological understanding of imagination. For a phenomenological approach, imagination is an act of experiencing something as possible rather than actual or present (Jansen 2010). Although imagination is understood as an act and, thus, involving human agency, it is not always voluntary or conscious. Rather it can be involuntary and occurring independently of conscious awareness, as Csordas describes it when referring to the spontaneity of imagination. Importantly, imaginary experience has a sensory content that makes it similar to the experience of perceiving (ibid.). Nevertheless, we are usually able to differentiate between imagined and perceived objects, except in pathological conditions, such as hallucinations. What makes imagination different to perceiving is that, whereas in perception objects appear as actual, in imagination objects appear as only possible (ibid.). In this way, phenomenologically understood, imagination is not only the visualization of mental images but the actual experience, through a sensory engagement, of possible (although not actual or present) objects or situations.

In the context Csordas studied, that of Catholic Charismatics in the U.S., imagination is performatively elaborated mostly through "imagery" or "visualization." A healer's account of how she inculcates visualization is compelling. It shows how Catholic Charismatic healers promote imagery as a mode of self-process, inculcating the capacity to visualize in patients. At the same time, it shows the performative efficacy of imagery.

> I give a "shoe test" to help people to visualize, to show them what I mean by visualization. I just tell them close your eyes … "Now, with your eyes closed I want you to picture a shoe. Okay, open your eyes." Now, I ask questions. Is it a man's shoe? Is it a woman's shoe? Does the shoe have buckles, laces, a slip-on? Is it the left shoe or the right shoe? [Etc.] And now this is where the audience calls out, right? I'll go like this and they call out "black," "brown," "white," "red," "pink," nyab, nyab, nyab. And then I'll say, "Okay, how many saw a tennis shoe, a sneaker, or jogging shoes, a wooden shoe, a

> glass slipper, a baby's shoe, a tap shoe, a toe shoe, a leprechaun's shoe, an Arabian shoe, a boot, a slipper, a doctor's shoe, a nurse's shoe, a surgical shoe, seventeenth century French cavalier boots, the Pope's shoe, a horseshoe, a policeman's shoe, a military shoe, combat boots?" And the hands are going up. When they're all finished I say [to] those that don't see, "You need a healing of your imagination." And I tell them why, because their creativity and their spontaneity were stifled as children. So we take Jesus back in their lives, and ask Jesus to heal all that hurt and trauma so they can visualize. "Now you people that saw a shoe, you too need a healing. You need to forgive the person whose shoe you saw." Ha! Ha! And this is where the audience goes, "Oh!" I'll say, "How many saw their own shoe?" Half the audience! I say, "You have to forgive yourself."
>
> (Csordas 1994a: 76)

In the example above, the shoe is a symbol of oneself or a significant other. At the same time, the shoe as a personal symbol emerges in performance through imagination (in this case through a concrete form of imagination: imagery or visualization). The images of the shoes "present" an existential situation and, at the same time, the different kinds of shoes "represent" a cultural meaning (Csordas 1994a: 81). In this way, Csordas proposes the complementarity between semiotics and phenomenology by claiming that "imagery is intelligible insofar as it inheres in the symbolic or semiotic order, and is efficacious as a self-process insofar as it inheres in the existential order of being in the world" (ibid.: 81). While the empiricist conceives of imagination as a mental object, phenomenology understands it as a modality of consciousness (ibid.: 80). Thus, there is a competing epistemological understanding of imagination that makes an empiricist and a phenomenological account of imagination incompatible. Instead, Csordas claims that the epistemological understanding of imagination between a semiotic and a phenomenological approach is not competing. Rather, both approaches account for a complementarity of imagination in the orders of representation and being in the world (ibid.: 80). For reconciling a phenomenological approach of imagination as "image in consciousness" with a semiotic approach of the image as sign, Csordas draws on Peirce's semiotics and Sartre's phenomenology (ibid.: 84–87).[2]

Hsu (2010: 353) noted that various anthropologists have acknowledged the possibilities Peirce's semiotics provide when he described relations of meaning that are non-symbolic (i.e., relations of meaning that are not generated by convention but by similarity and contiguity). Kohn (2007, 2013), drawing on Peirce, postulated that symbolic reference is constructed out of more basic non-symbolic sign processes that are common to all forms of living organisms. Therefore, semiosis is always embodied, and it is always entangled with material processes. The former ideas are in line with a phenomenological understanding of relations of meaning as grounded in the body (and, thus, always entangled with material processes).[3]

Csordas, also drawing on Peirce's semiotic, postulated that the images of the shoes have a content that acts as a "representamen," an object that is the person or situation that they represent and an interpretant "constituted by an explanation of the situation, a course of action to be taken in resolution of the problem, or an outcome in the form of a goal to be achieved in the healing process" (Csordas 1994a: 85).

Csordas proposes to use Sartre's understanding of imagination as complementary to Peirce's semiotics to account for the experiential engagement of a sign. In Sartre's account, imagination is an act that occurs in different sensory modalities and has a culturally specific form. Sartre's image also has an immediate content of consciousness that corresponds to Peirce's "representamen," and an object, such as a situation or problem. What is missing in Peirce's semiotics is the act, while in Sartre the interpretant is missing. In this way, performative efficacy relies on the understanding of a visual image and other concrete forms of imagination as an act (something that the body does). At the same time, the cultural meaning of a visual image depends on the existence of an interpretant. While performative efficacy of visual images accounts for experiential transformations of bodily and affective states, the cultural interpretation of visual images account for the understanding of a problematic situation and the reflexive exploration of possible solutions.

> The sign in itself has no act phase because, as a function of textuality, it is always already in the order of representation rather than of presentation, always primarily related to other signs and only secondarily to motives. Conversely, as a function of embodiment, the image in itself can have no definitive interpretant in the world …
>
> (Csordas 1994a: 86)

To clarify Csordas' proposal of reconciling a phenomenological and semiotic approach, I provide an ethnographic case about revelatory images among Catholic Charismatics in the U.S. (Csordas 1994a: 47). Revelatory images are spontaneous experiences of inspiration that are considered to be "spiritual gifts." Some of the most frequent cultural forms in which revelations occur are word of knowledge, word of wisdom, and vision or imagery. Word of knowledge consists of receiving information through divine inspiration, while word of wisdom is being able to say what a patient needs to hear. Vision or imagery consists in visualizing an image that can give significant information regarding a patient's situation. Contrary to word of knowledge and word of wisdom, which are only experienced by healers, both healers and patients can experience imagery. Revelatory experiences occur in the form of nonverbal sensory experiences in different modalities, such as visual images, haptic, kinesthetic and proprioceptive sensations, and affective sensations. These experiences constitute the pre-reflexive beginning of self-processes and constitute Sartre's conceptualization of imagination as an act. For Sartre (2004), the content of consciousness is an act because consciousness is intentional and directed toward others. Moreover, imagining an object is not only a simulacrum of the real object but the presentation, through a physical or affective experience, of the object in its corporeality.

Csordas conducted a rigorous ethnographic description of the image as an act in the context of Catholic Charismatic's revelatory gifts. These gifts occur in specific sensory modalities and cultural form. Visual imagery predominates among the Charismatics and it usually appeared "in the form of mental pictures, often of a person or situation, but sometimes of an afflicted body part, and occasionally as a number or word inscribed, as it were, on the tabula rasa of the mind" (Csordas 1994a: 89). Images based on the sense of touch were second in frequency. Under this category, Csordas grouped haptic, kinesthetic, and proprioceptive sensations. Some of the sensations reported were heat, pain, coldness, lightness or heaviness, burning, and electricity moving through the body. Other types of imagery modality were less frequent, such as auditory or olfactory. Because imagination is an act in which specific sensory and affective experiences are performatively elaborated, imagined images can become engaged as an existential reality.

Revelatory images fall into two categories of relationships between "representamen" and object described by Peirce (Csordas 1994a: 95–102). Revelatory images can be symbolic signs, and as such in need of an intellectual concept to link them to an object, or they can have a direct link to their object: icon and index in Peirce's terminology. Index and icon, then, are directly linked to an object without the necessity of conceptual analysis. An index directly links a "representamen" and its object due to contiguity. An icon directly links a "representamen" and its object due to similarity.

> Among the Charismatic healers in the present study, roughly half the images reported (N = 146) are symbolic signs of persons and situations, the interpretants of which are revelations about a patient's problem. The other half (N = 141) are indices or icons of a patient's state, the interpretants of which are revelations about the pragmatics of the ongoing healing event. Within the Charismatic cultural context, the latter are relatively self-evident in meaning and lack the condensation of meaning characteristic of symbols.
>
> (Csordas 1994a: 96)

According to the relationship between "representamen" and object there are four different types of "representamen" in Catholic Charismatic revelatory images. First, revelatory images can be indexical icons. For example, an emotional image experienced by a healer indicates the existence of an emotion in the afflicted and is, thus, an index. At the same time, the emotional image has the same form of that emotion and functions, thus, as an icon. Secondly, revelatory images can be indexes. Indexical images can be placed in a continuum of diminished iconicity (Csordas 1994a: 98). For example, the haptic image of physical warmth is an indexical icon of divine power in which warmth is equivalent to energy. Also, the haptic image of physical warmth localized in the feet and legs can be taken as an indexical revelation of a circulatory problem in which the sensation of warmth is indicating the location of a problem. Let us provide another example using the revelatory image of pain experienced by a healer. Pain in the ears of a healer is an indexical icon indicating a patient's ear problem. Pain bears an iconic relation with illness, and the location of pain is indexical to the location of the problem. While pain in the ears of a healer has both iconic and indexical elements, a healer's ear becoming red and flushed is a more purely indexical sign that God wants to speak.

Thirdly, revelatory images can be purely iconic. Common iconic revelatory images are the face or hands of Jesus (or other divine figures). Lastly, "representamens" can be symbolic signs such as the images of people, divine figures, objects, words or numbers, emotions, and impulses. Symbolic images require that healer and patient constitute the relationship between "representamen" and object as this relationship is not immediate and intuitive. Thus, symbolic images require an interpretant (Csordas 1994a: 101).

The possible alternatives of interpretants or explanations to symbolic revelatory images are provided by the habitus, which provides both the possible "representamens" and the possible interpretants that can be related to a particular problem or situation (Csordas 1994a: 106). In the context of Catholic Charismatics in the U.S., common interpretations to symbolic revelatory images are problems of intimacy, trauma, physical illness, emotional distress, spiritual problems, and sins. The semiotic element is given by the type of sign in which particular revelatory image occurs. For instance, the more ambiguous image of a fetus (an iconic sign) could have multiple interpretations such as trauma, sin, or relational difficulties. In contrast, the symbolic image of the word abortion written on an imaginal blackboard is more restrictively interpreted as a sin in the conservative worldview of the Catholic Charismatics. In this way, "the habitus regulates improvisation by defining the limits of reality, and semiosis regulates improvisation by defining the limits of specificity in revelatory imagery" (ibid.: 106).

It is noteworthy that revelatory images are constituted as symbols, icons or indexes according to their relationship with the object they represent. In other words, revelatory images are not inherently symbolic or non-symbolic, rather the way they are linked to an object depends on the context. In this way, the same sensorial experience can constitute symbolic or non-symbolic relations of meaning in accordance with the interpretation process. Thus, all relations of meaning are grounded in the body.

I have stated that Csordas' theory of self provides a rationale for understanding the mutual relations between symbolic and non-symbolic healing transformations. Imagination is the vehicle through which self-transformations occur in ritual healing. Imagination, phenomenologically understood, is an act that the body does, usually with a sensory modality and a cultural form. In this way, imagination can become experientially engaged and performed. At the same time, symbolic and non-symbolic relations of meaning culturally pattern the content of imagination. Therefore, a semiotic and a phenomenological approach can be deemed complementary when accounting for healing transformations.

In conclusion, we cannot restrict the understanding of healing transformations to purely symbolic transformations. By doing so we risk relying on overly broad and simplistic terms to understand healing efficacy and ignoring the effect sophisticated techniques have on people's bodies. Therefore, I have tried to complement the understanding of healing transformations as being only rearrangement in the relations between abstract concepts. In doing so, I relied on the body and the sensory and affective transformations the body experiences when exposed to healing techniques. Sensory experience, affective states and bodily habits provide the experiential ground to meaningful experience. Thus, for rearrangements of symbolic meaning to be experientially significant, they need to be achieved through the engagement of the body and its practices and skills.

Notes

1. In this section, I elaborate on Hsu's (2015) series of lectures in the option paper 'Sensory Experience in Therapeutics,' Oxford University.
2. The relation between these two orders of experience, namely the order of the body and the order of the text (Berger 1987), has been the object of anthropological concern and theorization. Other authors (e.g., Kirmayer 1992) postulated that metaphors, due to their embodied nature, can create meaning not only through representation but also through "enactment" or "presentation." Thus, metaphors can be both cognitive tools to rearrange concepts and create new meanings, and communicative acts constrained by social structure (ibid.: 337).
3. However, there are fundamental differences in the way Kohn (2007, 2013) and Csordas (1994a) understand representation and the semiotic order. While for Csordas representation is dependent on the human ability of reflexivity, Kohn postulates that the capacity for representation is shared by all living organisms (and is, then, not dependent on human reflexivity). In the same vein, Kohn rejects the dichotomy text/performance, which remains central in Csordas' proposition of a complementarity between phenomenology and semiotics.

Chapter 2
A Real Machi
Pewtun *and* Nguillatun *Rituals*

Among my interlocutors, doubts about whether a machi is a real machi were common. When I told my friends I wanted to learn about machi medical techniques they immediately warned me about avoiding "fake" or "bad" machi: "You need to be sure she is a real machi," I was advised many times. These doubts may refer to the suspicion of a machi really being a *kalku* (witch). Thus, a real machi is expected to use their powers to do good, whereas a *kalku* is someone who uses their powers to harm other people, either for money, envy, or revenge. Nevertheless, ambiguity is ever present, since a machi's powers can be used either to do good or to harm. In addition, witchcraft is not the only source of ambiguity with regard to a machi's powers. A machi's *pülli* (lineage spirit) is considered inherently unpredictable and revengeful, and people are afraid of what may happen if they inadvertently offend a machi's spirit. Moreover, machi need to be in permanent contact with *wekufe* (evil spirits) (S: *demonio*) or *wezanewen* (evil energies) to keep them at bay. When dealing with evil spirits, common human flaws, such as laziness, recklessness, and dishonesty, may have catastrophic consequences. Although many of my interlocutors framed the dichotomy between machi and *kalku* as "real" and "not real" machi, others put it as "good" machi and "bad" machi; that is, machi who do good and machi who harm their patients.[1]

The moral ambiguity of a machi's powers was not the only anxiety driving doubts about who is a real or good machi. In fact, it was probably not the most important one. Before choosing a machi, people need to know whether they really are a powerful shaman. In other words, whether they can really know and treat illness and misfortune. When my interlocutors were asked how they know if a machi is a good machi, both in moral terms and in their capacity for treating people effectively, the answer was pragmatic and simple. If a machi gives you *lawen* (remedies) that make you feel better, if they perform healing ceremonies that alleviate your symptoms, they are a real machi. In a context otherwise characterized by a conservative worldview, influenced by Catholicism and, more recently, other forms of Christianity, people can be very tolerant regarding machi's social conduct and status. For instance, popular machi can be men, women or transsexual women; old or young; uneducated or professionals; married, divorced or having public extramarital affairs; known problematic drinkers; Mapuche or people with mixed origins; political activists; and more. What people expect from machi is the capacity to know illnesses and misfortunes and provide treatment. Patients usually expect the machi to "see" the illness or problem through different diagnostic techniques or to be told about the problem by spirits, typically, in dreams and ritual trance. A patient can only know a machi "sees" the sickness when the machi names it. In addition, patients can only know the problem has been solved when they feel better, after receiving treatment.

In this chapter, I explore how to know who is a real machi in terms of their capacity to effectively see, treat, and prevent illness and misfortune. The power to treat cannot be entirely separated from a machi's moral constitution (i.e., whether they are a witch). Thus, machi who can effectively treat sick people are the ones chosen to preside over *ngillatun* rituals, which, in turn, reduces the moral ambiguity of the machi's powers.[3] Here, I ethnographically explore the way a Mapuche shaman, Machi Carmen, effectively diagnoses and treats her patients and is recognized by her community and others as a real machi. I have chosen Machi Carmen because she can be considered a successful shaman. She treats patients both in institutionalized and non-institutionalized settings. She is popular among rural and urban Mapuche, and among rural and urban non-Mapuche. In fact, people were coming to see her from different cities in the country, such as Santiago, Iquique and Concepción, and from Mapuche rural communities in Argentina. Moreover, she is a leader in her community, where she presides over the *ngillatun* ritual. She also presides over *ngillatun* rituals in communities different to her own. Although the cases described here correspond to the practice of one machi, I also provide general descriptions originated from the observations of other machis' practices, both in institutionalized and non-institutionalized settings, and in the context of the *ngillatun* ritual.

By ethnographically exploring the practice of a popular machi, I intend to theoretically revisit the problem of treatment effectiveness. Here, I understand treatment effectiveness as ritually induced transformations of the self (Csordas 1994a). I am interested in the reciprocity between aspects of those transformations occurring at a level that is pre-reflexive or prior to conscious awareness, and aspects occurring at a reflexive level. Here, my focus is on techniques that seek to predispose the subject to new dispositions to experience. After the subject has opened to change, ritual healing techniques organize sensorial and affective transformations through ritual action.

I start by providing a general contextualization of Machi Carmen's practice as a Mapuche shaman. Then, I describe how Machi Carmen can see and treat illness through a technique called *pewtun* or uroscopy. In discussing *pewtun* techniques, I aim to illustrate two issues. First, *pewtun* is a technique that seeks to promote the patient's imaginative engagement with the machi and the therapeutic procedure. Secondly, *pewtun* seeks to promote and intensify the emergence of affective forces that can engage the patient in a creative construction of meaning.

In the second part of the chapter, I explore the role of Machi Carmen as the presiding ancestral authority of a *ngillatun* ritual. The effective performance of *ngillatun* rituals reduces the moral ambiguity of the machi, enhancing their reputation as a powerful shaman. In addition, it gives an opportunity for the exchange of feelings of belonging and shared self-worth. In this way, Machi Carmen can strengthen her role as a health person, preventing sickness and natural disasters through her ability to enter *küymin* (ritual trance) and deliver a message from the spirits to the community. Also, she can heighten her role in community building and transmission of cultural practices.

A Real Machi

Machi Carmen is a middle-aged woman. She lives in a rural Indigenous community in the costal area of the Araucanía region. Machi Carmen treats patients at home and in different institutional settings. She travels once a week to a nearby town where she works in the Mapuche medical center. When she gets to the Mapuche medical center, there are usually at least thirty patients waiting for a consultation and another twenty to thirty people waiting to receive *lawen* (remedies) prescribed in past consultations. These numbers are clearly above the average of the rest of the machi (five in total) working there. Typically, a machi treats around ten patients per day and the staff at the Mapuche medical center distribute herbal infusions or *lawen* among ten to twenty more patients. In addition, Machi Carmen travels to various rural medical posts, located relatively close to her home, to treat patients and distribute the herbal infusions she produces at home. For all her institutionalized activities she receives a salary from the state (either from municipalities or from the Ministry of Health's regional office). For her eight hours per week job at the Mapuche medical center, she receives 500,000 Chilean pesos a month (US$830).[3] This is much higher than the minimum wage, which is 276,000[4] Chilean pesos (US$458) a month for forty-four hours a week (a full-time job). A general physician working full time (44 hours a week) in a primary care setting earns an average of 800,000 to 1,000,000 Chilean pesos (US£1,328 to 1,660) a month. Thus, Machi Carmen is significantly wealthier than those around her. Her wealth comes, to a significant extent, from her work at state health institutions, and it plays a significant role in accentuating her shamanic powers. Having said this, it is also true that, during my fieldwork, Machi Carmen was significantly more popular than other shamans who were as wealthy as she was (and who also worked in state institutions). Although wealth and state recognition do contribute to a machi having a good reputation, they do not entirely explain a machi's success. Moreover, I observed that working for state institutions can also be a source of distrust and criticism.

Machi Carmen prepares herbal infusions at home and she takes them to the Mapuche medical center in large plastic containers (each containing about twenty liters). Using these large containers, many individual bottles, of about a liter capacity, can be filled to provide remedies for many patients. Some machi can bring with them more than twenty different infusions, some for drinking, some for bathing. Machi Carmen is specially known because she brings a considerable number of different herbal infusions. Also, she brings different herbal infusions every week because she knows, through her dreams, what her patients will need. Nevertheless, other machi only bring two types of infusions: one for treating illnesses, *lawen* or remedies, and a second one as a counterhex (S: *contra*). Some friends did not trust any machi who provide treatment in Mapuche medical centers, because they thought they were giving the same remedy to every person: 'Just like doctors who give *paracetamol* (acetaminophen) to everybody,' a woman told me. Each plastic container is marked by a number, combination of numbers, letters, or combination of letters, which differ from one machi to the other. Machi do this so the staff at the health center, who are dispensing the herbal infusions to patients, know which one to give to each person. Machi do not reveal what the infusions contain, and nobody asks them because it is machi *kimün* (ancestral knowledge). Machi *kimün* can only be used for good purposes in the hands of a machi. However, people do understand general uses of numbers and letters after working for a while with a specific machi. In the case of Machi Carmen, she made an incredible number of different infusions, usually adding new herbs to a preparation for each specific patient (or telling the patient which herb he/she should add to the infusion she was giving them). Nevertheless, she had some preparations that she used repeatedly; for example, number one for urinary system problems, number two for depression, number five cleans the body inside, number eight for impaired vision, and "the bitter infusion" (S: *amargo*) for improving circulation and blood pressure. In addition, she always prepared infusions of mixed herbs that were considered counterhexes, such as rue and wormwood. Counterhex infusions should be used for bathing, not for drinking.

Currently, more and more patients are going to public Mapuche medical centers to be treated by a machi. However, many people prefer to go to a machi's home. The most significant difference is that at medical centers patients do not have to pay because the state (either through the regional office of the Ministry of Health or local municipalities) is paying the machi and all the staff. Contrarily, when going to a machi's house, patients need to pay. The cost varies significantly according to different machi. In addition, most machi charge patients differently according to what they perceive to be their economic circumstances; that is, they charge more to people from the city, professionals, and people coming from different Indigenous communities to their own. Overall, prices for a consultation range from a voluntary donation to 40,000 Chilean pesos (about US$60). Machi Carmen does not charge friends and relatives but rather asks for a voluntary donation. It is not unusual for people to decide to pay her large sums of money, as it is considered a fair compensation (to fairly compensate the machi is considered necessary for recovery). Another significant difference between institutionalized and non-institutionalized consultations is that machi usually give more time to patients in their homes. While institutionalized consultations rarely last more than twenty minutes, it is usual for a machi to stay longer (even several hours) with a patient in their home. Moreover, if the patient is also a friend (which is very common) he/she could be invited to stay to share a meal and *mate* tea, an invitation that would be considered rude to refuse without a good excuse.

Consultations start around eight in the morning and they stop at midday (though in institutional settings they continue until the machi has treated all the patients). It is thought that machis' powers to see illnesses are stronger in the morning. As machi attend patients according to the order of arrival, people tend to arrive very early, waiting together for the machi to start working and call them one by one. Every machi I knew living in rural areas (six in total) lived in a modern house that was, in some cases, a state-subsidized house. There are special subsidies for Mapuche shamans, who can apply to get larger houses than other people. This is locally justified by the fact that patients commonly spend the night at the shaman's house when a special healing ceremony called the *ulutun* ritual is performed. Thus, machi need extra space so their patients can spend the night at their homes. Machi Carmen's house is much larger than the average house. It has two floors and a bathroom (many houses do not have bathrooms and people use latrines). Her house was built using her own financial resources, without state subsidies.

The traditional Mapuche houses or *ruka* are no longer used as homes, but machi still perform their consultations and some ceremonies inside them. Thus, what is common to see in a machi's home today, as in the case of Machi Carmen, is a modern house, of varying size, and next to it a traditional Mapuche house or *ruka* with its door facing east. A *ruka* is a round building with a conical roof. The walls are built using native wood and *coligüe* rods, which is a species of bamboo. The roof is covered with *junquillo*, straw, or some similar type of grass. The *rewe* or altar is usually facing the *ruka*'s door.[5] The *rewe* is a trunk of native wood that has been carved. It has several steps that lead to a tip with an anthropomorphic face. It is usually adorned with branches of native trees, such as *canelo* (canelo), *maitén* (mayten) and *maqui* (Chilean wineberry), among others, as well as flags of different colors. Machi put the urine (bottled in plastic or glass containers) or clothing of their patients on the steps of the *rewe* and leave it there until the old branches of native trees are removed and replaced by new branches. The renewal of the *rewe* is performed in a ceremony called the *ngeikurewen* ritual, which is done every year (although the frequency varies from one machi to the other). Thus, the patient continues to receive the positive effects of the machi's *llellipun* (prayers), even though they might not be physically in contact. Machi perform their *llellipun* every morning, before sunrise, playing their *kultrun* (ritual drum) and chanting.

"Seeing" Illnesses and Misfortunes: *Pewtun* Techniques

The most frequent method of divination nowadays is a technique called *pewtun* (a word deriving from the Mapudungun verb root *pen*, which means to see).[6] The technique consists of the visual inspection of the patient's urine (the first one of the day) that has been previously bottled in a transparent plastic or glass container. It could also be done by looking at the patient's clothing or photographs. Today, it is more common to use the patient's bottled urine, which is a specific type of *pewtun* called *willentun*. Bacigalupo (2001, 2007) previously described uroscopy as a popular technique among machi. Her observations were based on extensive fieldwork in the 1990s. I observed that uroscopy has become the most popular divinatory technique by far. The machi may decide to arrange more complex healing rituals according to what is seen in the urine. In most cases, they prescribe medicinal herbal infusions. Patients are frequently advised to come back for a checkup. It is not uncommon for some patients to keep coming for months or even years.

The technique appeared during the nineteenth century, probably influenced by the popularity of uroscopy in Europe (Stolberg 2015) and the import of Europeans' theory of humors (Bacigalupo 2001: 71). It has been replacing (although not entirely) other Mapuche divinatory techniques such as divination through the inspection of internal organs of ritually sacrificed animals or divination by drumming over the patient's clothing (Bacigalupo 2007). The growing number of Mapuche public medical centers since the 2000s has contributed to the increasing popularity of the technique to the detriment of others. In institutionalized settings, it is the only technique used, and to bring a urine sample is a prerequisite to receive the service (although sometimes a machi may accept it if the patient provides his/her clothing instead of the urine). Uroscopy is cheaper, simpler and more adaptable to institutionalized settings than other techniques. Thus, the technique allows incipient practices of state bureaucratization of machi medical practices.

Most of my friends insisted that machi should see the urine (S: *ver la orina*). However, when asked what machi are supposed to see, most people were puzzled. They were not referring to forms, colors or textures. Rather, when they said they expected the machi to see, they were saying they expected the machi to know or understand: 'to know what is going on with me,' (S: *que sepa lo que me pasa*) a friend told me. Therefore, they were referring to the spiritual capacity of a machi to recognize an illness or problem when seeing the urine. That is to say that they expected the machi to divine the disease or to be aware of the problematic circumstances they were facing. Only after knowing could the machi prescribe remedies and advise their patient. To prove they can really see the urine, a machi must know what is wrong with the patient without her/him telling her. The insistence of my friends that the machi must prove that they see appeals to the veracity and credibility of the diagnosis/divination.

Machi Carmen once told me that a friend of hers who is a doctor told her that he could also see the urine. His statement initially surprised her, as only shamans or people with spiritual gifts can do that. But when the doctor explained what he could see, she was amused. He said: "I can see whether it is turbid or clean, or if it has blood or pus," Machi Carmen told me. She laughed when saying this. Evidently, this is not what she can see in the urine. But when trying to explain what it is that she can see, she had trouble finding the words. "It is not only what you see, but what you feel. If you feel a pain in the kidneys you need to pay attention to the kidneys," she tried to explain. It became clear to me that to see the urine was not limited to seeing images, colors, or shapes in it, as the doctor stated. Rather, it was a sensory experience involving feeling and seeing with the whole body. In addition, as I will describe below, to see the urine is a relational process involving input from an active patient.

A typical *pewtun* (uroscopy) technique occurs in the following way. Machi and patient (commonly accompanied by family members) usually greet each other with a kiss on the cheek, between women and men or between two women, or with a hand clasp in the case of two men. The duration of the greeting is, in general, short but courteous and affectionate, especially when people already know each other. Asking about the health of family members is usual, even more so when those family members are also patients (and friends) of the machi. Patients also ask for the state of health of the machi and their family. Both machi and patient sit facing each other, usually with a table between them. On the table it is common to see 10,000-peso notes and *foye* (canelo) leaves. Family members usually sit behind the patient or next to her/him.

The patient passes the container with the urine to the machi either in the hand or places it on the table. Then, the machi usually takes the container to stare at it from different angles, sometimes shaking it. Little verbal interchange occurs at the beginning, and most patients wait patiently for the machi to start speaking. The time the machi takes to stare at the urine varies greatly from one case to the other. This moment of the encounter is significant because it is how the machi can direct the patient's attention. By staring at the urine, the machi generates a moment of synchronicity (Hsu 2005) in which both machi and patient direct their attention to the same object and experiential situation. Therefore, great expectation is generated as to what the machi might see in the urine. Usually, this is a tense moment. It is not uncommon for patients to be afraid about what the machi may see. This is especially the case when people fear they might have been the victims of black magic (something that machi commonly divine). Thus, staring at the urine sample is a technique that seeks to actively engage the patient with the situation, predisposing him/her to imaginatively open up to new possible interpretations.

When the machi starts speaking about what they are seeing in the urine, they tend to make little eye contact, staring either at the urine or staring elsewhere, without apparent aim. What usually follows next is that the machi describes the patient's symptoms, such as headache or stomachache, or conditions such as weakness of the blood, affecting different organs, parts, and systems of the body. There is frequently an order followed from head to foot, although this is not always the case. The machi engages in a type of speech that is inconsistent, contradictory, and open to interpretation. Many symptoms are enunciated, as well as descriptions of the life circumstances of a person, such as problems at work or with the family. Most of these enunciations are not further discussed and do not become the central issue of the consultation. The patient actively participates with both verbal and nonverbal interventions, guiding the machi in choosing some aspects of their enumeration of problems and abandoning others. Some patients do not speak, either because they feel it is disrespectful or because they want proof that the machi can know what is wrong without them telling them. Even if they do not speak, they participate in the form of nods and expressions of approval or disapproval. Others are more prone to verbally guiding the machi to the issue they want to address. In most cases patients act somehow in between, which is to say they provide some verbal explanations, but only after the machi has said something to elicit it. When machi and patient have reached an agreed upon topic together, the initial inconsistent monologue of the machi changes into a coherent dialogue between machi and patient (and sometimes this includes the patient's family members). In this way, machi and patient can identify a problem and what is required to overcome it.

Machi speech parallels the description of what Parkin (1991) called "jumbled speech" in the context of Kenyan diviners. "Jumbled speech" is an "inconsistent and mixed use of metaphors, false syllogism, some reversals, and an apparent lack of path control" (ibid.: 185): "Jumbled ideas and metaphors that suggest various possible interpretations give way to their ordered sequencing and to more limited interpretations; they are finally superseded by an unambiguous classification of the causes of the sickness and the material needed to cure it" (ibid.: 183).

Although some resolution and consensus about a diagnosis do occur, Parkin's approach may appear too simple. In fact, the machi divinations tend to be more ambiguous than the Kenyan cases that Parkin described. The divinations may be incomplete, and the patient may require further procedures; the main divination may change within a single consultation; previously abandoned themes can be taken up again in a single consultation or through various encounters; and machi usually advise to come back if the problem persists, leaving open the possibility that the treatment may not be enough. Thus, the process of divining is never completely ended and there is always the possibility of a next step. Geissler and Prince's (2010) concept of "trying out" may complement and expand Parkin's approach. When discussing the practices mothers in Western Kenya use to treat their sick children, they realized that treating and trying medicines was more important than reaching a specific diagnosis:

> Various potential illnesses were discussed, but it remained unclear (indeed, unimportant at this point) what the child's "real" problem was; a range of medicines was suggested, and few were tried out immediately. In addition, the chronology of illness and treatment was unclear: there was no clear beginning and even weeks later, after a visit to the health post and treatment for malaria, there was no conclusion.
>
> (Geissler and Prince 2010: 212)

Thus, by "trying out," people permanently seek a definite understanding of a problem that never arrives. Rather, they keep moving forward with "possibilities and opportunities for action" (Geissler and Prince 2010: 212). "Trying out" is not the same as "trial and error." The former "acknowledges contingency and the absence of control" (ibid.: 204), while the latter understands the "relation between person, tool and task … [as] constituted by instrumental intentionality" (ibid.: 204). The *pewtun* ritual I am describing here is a formal diagnostic/divinatory ritual, while mothers caring for their children constitute informal, everyday practices. Thus, it is not surprising that machi practices are more constricted by a body of expert knowledge. Also, patients do expect some resolution and understanding of their problems. Nevertheless, what is important to notice is that some ambiguity and lack of closure is always present. In this way, machi can "try out" new diagnoses in following consultations or different treatments, and patients may continue to play an active part, such as deciding to go to other machi or other type of practitioners.

The machi speech in the *pewtun* technique is a playful speech in the sense that it produces a subjunctive mode. In this way, the presence of an imprecise and open speech brings with it the potentiality of creating new forms of meaning. This is in line with anthropological endeavors aiming at reconceptualizing ritual and play as the construction of an "as if" world or a subjunctive world (Seligman et al. 2008: 17–42). In addition, the machi speech is a technique to promote the patient's imagination. Imagination refers to the creative capacity of reflexively changing one's disposition to the world. Also, when transformed into specific forms, imagination is a mode of self-processes (or a mode of constitution of the self) (Csordas 1994a: 74). Specific culturally patterned forms of promoting the imagination can be framed as "somatic modes of attention" (Csordas 1993). In the case of *pewtun*, the form of the machi speech can create an attentive and responsive client, who is then able to generate redefinitions of his/her experience.

The Student's Home Full of Evil Spirits

The following transcript is an interchange between a young woman and Machi Carmen in the machi's *ruka* (Mapuche traditional house). Inside, the *ruka* of Machi Carmen measured approximately twenty meters long, ten wide and three high (in the highest part). It is a very dark place because the open door is the only source of light. In general, the machi sits with her patients in front of the open door to have some light. The rest of the space inside the *ruka* is full of stacked tables and chairs. At the center of the *ruka* there is always a fire, both to heat and to illuminate the place. Although some machi prepare medicinal infusions using the fire in their *ruka*, Machi Carmen uses the kitchen of the house where she lives. Therefore, after each consultation she goes to her kitchen to prepare a medicinal infusion for the patient. She usually hires assistants (usually her daughter or close friends who receive pay in cash) who help her prepare the herbal infusions.

This consultation began with an unusually long silence. The machi was not only staring at the urine but also at the patient, who was a woman in her early twenties (younger than the usual patient). From the way she was dressed she seemed to be living in the city. The bottle in which she put the urine was a foreign brand of mineral water, a brand people can only find in Temuco, which is the closest city. The silence was uncomfortable. I remember feeling nervous about the machi's long silence. The client seemed very nervous, even frightened. Her legs were constantly moving, she was pressing her purse against her thighs, and she did not establish eye contact.

The silence was finally broken by the machi asking a question. To start asking questions is not common for Machi Carmen. (In the transcript below I use M to indicate the machi is speaking and P to indicate the patient is speaking).

M: Where are you from?

P: From the town [She meant the local town. She did not live in an Indigenous rural community.]

M: Have you come before?

P: No.

M: Have you been using cards? [She meant tarot.]

P: No.

M: Do you study, do you work? [Again, these types of questions are not the usual thing.]

P: I study at the university.

There was another long silence. The machi continued to stare at the urine, took the bottle and started looking at it from different angles. She then put it back on the table between her and the patient. By doing this, the machi accentuated the tension. As was stated above, the initial part of the technique, in which the machi stares at the urine, seeks to direct the attention of the client, completely engaging them with the situation and building up expectations as to what the machi is going to say.

M: I want to know when it was that you fell asleep and then you woke up and you could not fall asleep again?

The machi asked this question with authority, demonstrating the confidence she had in that what she was asking had actually happened. The patient's response was immediate.

> *P:* Two nights ago. Where I live, I don't get any sleep.
>
> *M:* Yes, I saw that, I was surprised.

Machi Carmen re-signified her initial perplexity. This episode shows how a skillful machi can use her own affective experiences in at least two ways. First, she is generating a sense of empathy: she can understand what the patient is going through. Second, she seemed to be claiming that she actually saw what was going on in the urine. Thus, the divination was reliable.

> *P:* Before, there lived a young man who experimented with cards [she meant tarot] in the house I'm living now. We talked to him last week and he said he had taken the evil spirit out of the house. [The patient explained she lived in a Mapuche students' home in Temuco during the week. Several other students lived in the same house. She went home to her husband and child at weekends.]
>
> *M:* The house is full of spirits and your aura is very sensitive. As you do not sleep at all you are very sad, melancholic, sensitive, everything affects you. You watch TV and you suffer when you see someone suffering.
>
> *P:* I feel enormous pressure in my studies. [The patient cried. She went on to explain how difficult it is to study and be a mother and a wife at the same time.] I'm the last generation in my program at the university, after us it will no longer be offered.[7]

The initial affective state of the patient was anxiety and tension. However, when she began to talk about issues other than the presence of evil spirits in her house, the predominant emotion was sadness. The machi listened, establishing eye contact and showed interest. It was the machi who introduced sadness as a possibility by saying to the patient she was sad. In saying that, the machi gave an opportunity to talk about the difficulties the patient was facing. Although her difficulties of being a mother, wife, and student never became the central theme of the consultation, to talk about them produced a highly emotional moment.

M: There, they experimented with cards, candles and incense. [The machi is going back to the theme of evil spirits.]

P: Yes, that is what the young man said.

M: First, we must put a vase with honey and sugar on the dining table. With a white candle we make the spirits leave. The candle should be large, and you should light it at sunset, when the sun is going.

P: Where should I light it?

M: On the dining table.

P: I live in a student's home.

M: Yes, put water, sugar and honey on the dining table and into a vase. You are going to sweeten the water. Put any flower into the vase and put it on the table with the white candle next to it.

P: Why is this affecting me more than the others [students]? I'm going crazy.

M: Because you are too sensitive. I know you are not getting any rest. That is why I was looking at you; I was surprised.

P: I feel I brought bad energy [S: *mala energía*] from where I live in Temuco to my house here. My daughter did not sleep the other night.

M: You better do this in your house here.

P: But I live in Temuco.

M: It is chasing you, don't you see?

P: Really? On Friday, we talked with the young man. He will come back to the house because the other residents asked him to do something. He thinks he left the house clean and he wants to do it again.

M: Let him go. You must light your white candle and put salt next to it. Everything must be white, so it will be cleansing.

P: People told me I shouldn't do any counterhex because spirits get angry.

M: Yes, that young man left the spirits there. If someone grabs that aura, that person may even be driven to commit suicide. You need to bathe with *lawen* [remedies]: *ajenjo* [absinthe], *ruda* [rue], *romero* [rosemary], *triwe* [a native species of laurel] and *palo santo* [*Bursera graveolens*]. [The client writes down the names of the herbs.] You must boil all these herbs together and then add them to the infusion I will give you now. Then, you must take a bath.

P: In the bathtub?

M: As you wish. The young man is inexperienced, he is exploring, but he does not know. It is dangerous to go to the house, but they [the rest of the students who live in the house] are in the majority, and they will not listen to you. You can't convince the group [to not let the young man come back and try to expel the spirits]. So, you must take your bath and have your counterhexes. When the man comes you light your white candle and put salt next to it.

P: Can you see anything else?

M: Irritable bowel. That is due to stress.

P: Only stress?

M: Yes.

In this case, the machi makes use of nonverbal elements, such as silences and sharp looks at the urine and the patient, to generate an increase in tension and the reinforcement of negative affective states, mainly anxiety and sadness. The increase of an anxious affective state in the patient could be observed in the expression of her face and the movement of her body, especially the continuous rocking of her legs. In addition, I, as participant observer, could feel in my own body an increasingly unpleasant feeling, which engaged me with the situation and its possible ways of resolution. Then, the tension reached a climax, which the machi broke with the following question: 'I want to know when it was that you fell asleep and then you woke up and you could not fall asleep again?' This question is still an open question that could have had many answers. The patient was able to imaginatively answer the question as a way of reflexively engaging with her worries, but also as a way of reducing the anxiety that her body had been building up. Thus, after this question the tension was reduced. Following the reduction in the tension, a dialogue between machi and patient was constructed, in which the problem and the solution were discussed and agreed upon.

Although the dialogue constructed was mainly about the presence of evil spirits, other themes were also addressed. The patient worried about her roles as mother, wife and student. The reinforcement of negative affective states allowed the patient to address these concerns. In addition, she worried about her physical health. When the patient asked if her irritable bowel was only due to stress, she was asking whether she had any physical disease. Thus, when the machi answered that the symptoms were only due to stress, she was denying the presence of a serious physical disease.

The Woman Whom Nobody Loved Enough

In this case, it is observed that, in addition to a tentative and open speech, and the handling of looks, gestures, and silences to increase negative affective states, the machi uses a pre-constructed narrative capable of eliciting feelings of sadness. This narrative is based on prior knowledge of what kinds of narrative contents will elicit what kinds of emotions. Therefore, it requires a contextual knowledge, which, as we shall see, is a gendered knowledge.

The following case shows the interchange between Machi Carmen and a new patient in the machi's home. It was recorded on May 24, 2017. The machi took a small Coca-Cola bottle, containing the patient's urine, and stared at it for some seconds. The patient was a woman in her fifties.

M: Are you taking *wingka lawen* [Western medicine]?

P: One the midwife gave me.

M: Headache ... that happens sometimes.

P: Yes, but it is gone now.

M: An annoying feeling in the brain, it goes down to the shoulders and the back, and does it always reach the waist?

P: Yes, almost always.

M: This is when you are cold or when you are worried? [The patient hesitates to answer. The machi proceeds without waiting for the answer.] Altered nervous system, anxiety, preoccupations, fatigue. Swelling and weakening of bones [S: *ablandamiento de huesos*]. You have so many

> concerns, sadness. You feel nobody loves you, nobody values you. Sometimes you think about sleeping without ever waking up. [The client was crying, the machi handed her a tissue and continued, now establishing eye contact.] You work too much, like a man and like a woman [she meant the client performed both gender roles]. You feel sad because people do not value that. Sometimes people greet you, sometimes they act as if they had not seen you. You give it all away to them from your heart. You must go on because you do not have bad feelings, you are always giving to people and you do it with love.

Suddenly, the machi's speech changed from describing physical symptoms to describing suffering derived from unloving relationships. I was surprised at how quickly this narrative produced an easily observable emotional response in the client. It was literally so fast that I missed the beginning of it, by looking at the notebook where I was writing my notes for a couple of seconds. Although the machi's speech does not seem too long when transcribed, it actually lasted several minutes. The discordancy is probably due to some repetitions and a slow pace. In addition, in the English translation fewer words are required to convey the same idea. The intense moment produced was followed by a small pause. The machi and the patient looked at each other and both smiled. The patient stopped crying after that.

> *M:* You also have irritable bowel, which is due to stress.
>
> *P:* Yes. Is it only stress?
>
> *M:* Yes. And you do not sleep well. Sometimes you get up at night and you think and think [the patient nods]. Okay, darling [S: *ya, Mamita*] I will give you the *luwen* [remedies] you need.

The example shown above illustrates how a tentative speech generates an emotional response, which helps to transform that initial speech into a coherent narrative about emotional pain. The narrative about a woman's feelings of not being sufficiently valued by others is common in Machi Carmen's repertoire. For instance, she said the following to another female patient:

> You are always giving to others, with your hands full, giving all away, but sometimes you are giving a lot to people and you realize you are not being

> valued. Then, you say I will stop caring for this person. But you continue to be the same person. That saddens you, when you think why people don't acknowledge what I do for them. You give yourself away, you are always thinking about others, but who thinks about you?

It is frequent for this type of speech, focused on feelings of not being valued or loved, to produce an emotional response in the form of crying and sobbing. The machi do not use this type of narrative with men. When it comes to men, the machi points to a life of excessive physical work and hardship as the source of suffering. Men do not cry when exposed to this type of narrative, as this is stigmatized as feminine behavior. But, when confronted with the idea of having had to work too hard, the machi is usually able to elicit gestures of agreement and anecdotes about hard work and humiliating experiences. For instance, a man told the machi he was punched in the face by an army official during mandatory military service. After this incident, he was left with a persistent pain in his jaw. "Because we are poor, we must accept humiliations," he added. Thus, the machi knows the context and their knowledge is gendered. Using their knowledge, the machi can elicit memories of painful experiences both in men and women, promoting a fitting affective state and the involvement of the patient in the creation of a creative dialogue. The patient in the case above did not lead the machi through verbal interactions, rather her emotional response, in the form of crying, was a way of communicating an emotional state. The crying of the patient, in turn, can guide the speech of the machi. The machi has the capacity to put emotional suffering into words in a way that is meaningful to the patient.

The *pewtun* technique seeks to promote shared affective states, so that they can generate shared attentiveness and awareness in culturally specific ways. Notably, the feelings elicited are negative such as fear and sadness. This is in line with Hsu's (2005) observation about the role of acute pain in therapeutic encounters. Physical and emotional pain, when it is inflicted on a patient, with a demarcated beginning and end, can awaken and open the patient's body to the environment. In addition, as pain is accessed immediately through shared bodily experiences it can create a sense of connectedness and trans-individuality that is experienced as therapeutic. In other words, emotional pain can produce a shared somatic experience, in which everybody involved is grasped by the same affective state. Preconceived gendered narratives about emotional pain can be effective in generating intense shared emotional responses because people share the same habitus (Pandolfi 2007). That is to say that people have past knowledge that is embodied in a cultural history. The narrative used can, at the same time, predispose the client to new understandings and provides a meaningful narrative about emotional suffering.

The Man Who Frustrated the Machi

In the case that follows, I observed a patient's unwillingness to imaginatively engage with the machi's speech. That the diagnosis was so difficult can be attributed to a lack of imagination on the part of the patient or to the machi failing to promote it. It could also be due to the expectation that the machi can see the urine like a bone fracture is seen on an X-ray. In either case, what becomes apparent is that the patient is an active participant, rather than a passive receiver of a diagnosis. In other words, the machi cannot achieve a diagnosis without the participation of the patient. For this reason, if the patient is passively waiting for the machi to achieve a diagnosis, and withholds any kind of active engagement, diagnosis is severely affected.

The following is the dialogue between Machi Carmen and an 81-year-old male patient who did not know the machi previously. The consultation occurred in an institutionalized setting, specifically in the Mapuche medical center where Machi Carmen works.

> *M:* You have always had headaches … [She started speaking after staring at the urine for a couple of seconds.]
>
> *P:* Yes.
>
> *M:* Fatigue [S: *decaimiento*].
>
> *P:* No.
>
> *M:* Chill [S: *enfriamiento*], stomach gurgles [S: *crujimiento de estómago*].[8]
>
> *P:* Almost never.
>
> *M:* Pressure on the nervous system, blood pressure, prostate …

The different symptoms enunciated are not related. This is an illustrative case of the kind of open, tentative, and apparently aimless speech machis use.

> *P*: [Interrupting] I came for something that is urgent. I hope the disease I have will be shown in the urine.
>
> *M*: [Immediately continues her speech] You also have diabetes, that is why you are dizzy. You are also hungry. You eat but you are still hungry. Your vision has been declining, as well as your hearing. You also have blood pressure problems. You should not eat salt.
>
> *P*: Yes, yes … I know that. I also have the nerves [S: *también a uno le dan los nervios*].
>
> *M*: That is what I am telling you, your nervous system is altered. [She said this sounding irritated.] The urine also says you have an ulcer. All this comes due to lots of worries, because you work and work. [She tried to use a narrative about hardship and hard work that usually works well with her male clients.]
>
> *P*: I have not worked the land for seven years.

The answer above made me laugh (I had to hide my laughter because it would have been inappropriate). The patient was rejecting all of the machi's suggestions. The situation amused me in the same way a patient making a doctor look like a fool, with an argument against any possible diagnosis, would. It was evident that the patient was not doing it deliberately. Rather, he seemed to be genuinely looking for a true diagnosis, which did not coincide with the machi's speech.

> *M*: But your mind keeps on working, and all the work you used to do …
>
> *P*: Well yes, before it was like that. We, the Mapuche, had to work and work.
>
> *M*: That is what is producing consequences now. Despite everything you have gone through you are still alive. All you had to work … [The machi still tried to engage the patient into a narrative of hardship.]
>
> *P*: [Interrupting again] Sometimes, in the urine, it does not appear all. I would like all to be shown there.

M: Okay … the nails, there is something there, sometimes an itching.

P: Yes.

M: Problems in the left no … the right arm?

P: Yes, the right one.

M: Varicose veins.

P: Yes.

M: You must take care of your nails.

P: I have broken nails and they do not grow.

M: This is what I have to say *lamgen* [brother].

It appeared she was putting an end to the consultation. It was very unusual for Machi Carmen to do this without achieving a consensual diagnosis, which could have been an indication of her frustration. In fact, I had never observed her doing that before or since. Nevertheless, when she said, 'This is what I have to say,' she remained seated in the same position looking at the patient. Usually, when she was about to put an end to a consultation, she would stand up and walk outside her *ruka* to her house to prepare medicinal infusions. If the machi is in a Mapuche medical center, as in this case, she would end a consultation by writing a prescription on a piece of paper. With the prescription written, the patient would later go to the pharmacy to withdraw their medicinal herbal infusions. Finally, Machi Carmen decided to continue "trying out."

M: Did you ever have a big knock?

P: No.

M: Did you ever smoke?

P: When I was young.

M: The lungs seem in bad shape. You have everything swollen inside you. You must eat carefully and take care during this cold weather.

P: For the swollen prostate and all that, do I have a cure?

M: Yes, I will give you remedies. *Llantén* [*plantago major*] for the prostate and *quillay* [soapbark] for the lungs.

P: What if I tell you now what I have. Would that be good? Or should I keep it for myself?

M: You should tell me!

P: Last Friday, I had a pork *cazuela* [S: *cazuela de chancho*] for lunch [S: *almuerzo*]. Then, I had an *arrollado* [pork meat rolled in bacon with chili and spices] and a *manquehuito* [a popular national brand of white wine flavored with sugary soda]. After eating all this, my stomach starting aching [S: *me empezó a doler el estómago*] until I could not stop crying because of the pain.

M: I told you since the beginning you have stomach gurgles! [She tried to re-signify what she had said at the beginning of the consultation.]

P: I went to see a doctor and he told me I need to see him again today.

M: That is what I told you since the beginning: you have stomach gurgles! I will give you number 1, 5 and the bitter one [S: *amargo*]. [The patient is supposed to drink these three different types of herbal infusions.] You will take with you an infusion to take a bath with [S: *va a llevar un baño*]. And you will boil *matico* [orange-ball-tree]. Do you have *matico*?

P: Yes.

M: Okay. You must boil *matico, toronjil cuyano* [white horehound] and *lingue* [*persea lingue*]. You must add this to what I am giving you now to take a bath with. You should not drink it! You also need to add to this bath white vinegar and oregano.

The exchange described above was particularly difficult for the machi as it is unusual for a patient to expect such a specific diagnosis and to dismiss almost every word the machi said as close enough to his worries. Thus, the patient seemed rigidly expecting to hear what was already decided as the problem. Despite what one could frame as a lack of imagination on the part of the patient, the machi tried to recover trust. In this way, after the patient verbally constructed his problem, by himself, she tried to re-signify what she had already said at the beginning of their encounter: "You have stomach gurgles." In addition, she immediately went forward to provide prescriptions that could alleviate the patient's symptoms. Her attempts were at least partially successful. Although the patient was not entirely convinced his disease had been shown in the urine, he did seem convinced the machi knew how to cure him once he described his symptoms. The patient's willingness to follow the machi's prescriptions was evident in the fact that he asked the machi to write down the name of the herbs she was recommending.

For what has been described so far, the technique of *pewtun* could be detailed as follows. First, the inspection of the urine on the part of the machi generates tension and expectation. The patient's attention is completely focused on the machi's words and attitudes, which provides an opportunity to manipulate attention toward specific affective states and themes. Secondly, the machi's speech, both in its verbal contradictions and inaccuracies, and in its silences and gestures, promotes a creative patient willing to be an active participant in the complex, and usually fragmentary, creation of a problem and a solution. The initial speech of the machi does not intend to generate a coherent system of meaning, rather it aims at actively engaging the patient in an imaginative dialogue. Both the speech of the machi and the tense initial moment in which they stare at the urine, produce the circulation of shared affective states (Devisch 1990), as it was described in the first two cases. The different states that are elicited are usually negative, such as fear and sadness.

Each individual session of *pewtun* builds up a relationship of trust between machi and patient. Usually, a patient will recommend the machi who he/she trusts to family and friends. In addition, a trustful patient will continue to seek the help of the same machi. In this way, machi develop bonds of trust with a web of individuals and families who are, in turn, connected to each other. Moreover, machi can become the machi of an Indigenous community. In this role, machi do not only deal with illnesses and misfortunes but also preside over the *ngillatun* ritual (and other community ceremonies).

Ngillatun Ritual: Preventing Illness and Misfortune

Presiding over the *ngillatun* ritual enhances a machi's authority and prestige. In this way, people do not only differentiate who is a real machi according to their experiences with a machi in moments of crisis and illness. Rather, *ngillatun* ritual events (and other community ceremonies) are fundamental in creating a machi's pool of clients and social legitimacy. A machi who presides over the *ngillatun* ritual reduces the ambiguity of their powers.

The *ngillatun* ritual is the most important social and religious event in Mapuche rural life. It has been extensively studied by chroniclers and ethnographers since the sixteenth century.[9] My friends refer to it by using the words *ngillatun* or ceremony (S: *ceremonia*) interchangeably.[10] My friends explained to me that the *ngillatun* is a ceremony to offer thanks for what has been received and ask for good fortune. A friend told me: "The *ngillatun* is a spiritual purchase. I ask for something, but all the act of asking is what I give in return. And what I ask is to maintain the planet's equilibrium, from the person to the whole planet." Another friend told me that the *ngillatun* is the Mapuche way of communicating with God. Most people who participate in these ceremonies fear consequences if the ceremonies are not carried out. These consequences may be natural disasters, loss of the harvest, illness, and death.

A *ngillatun* ritual usually involves *llellipun* (prayers), *pürun* (ritual dancing) and animal sacrifice (usually a lamb). If a machi is the presiding ancestral authority, the ceremony also involves *küymin* (ritual trance). After a *ngillatun* is completed the participants gather around the *rewe* or altar to discuss the events that took place during the ceremony. The *ngillatun* ritual takes place twice a year, every two or four years, depending on different regions and communities. The first event (which is the biggest one) occurs in November or December, and the main goal is to ask for a good harvest and fertility. The second event takes place after the harvest during March or April. This second event is called the *kamarrikun* ritual and it is thought as a moment to thank for what was received during the summer or harvest period. The specific dates in which the ceremonies take place are usually determined by the *longko* (headman) together with a small group of men. On some occasions, a machi (or other ancestral authorities) can decide to conduct additional ceremonies, at different times of the year, in response to dreams or spirits' messages during trance. Only a very respected machi will be able to mobilize their community to perform this kind of ceremony. On one occasion, I participated in a ceremony that was carried out by a community from the mountains, about seventy miles to the east of where

Machi Carmen lived. They asked Machi Carmen to preside over the ceremony they wanted to perform to ask the *ngen* or spiritual guardian of a river to prevent the construction of a hydroelectric dam by a private company. Machi Carmen agreed to preside over that ceremony. Thus, Mapuche communities can decide to perform a *ngillatun* in moments of shared difficulties and hardship.[11]

The event I witnessed was carried out after Machi Carmen announced she had dreamt of illnesses and earthquakes. The community was not supposed to celebrate the *ngillatun* ritual that year because they do it only every four years. But, due to the machi's dream, they decided to conduct a *pichi* (small) *ngillatun*. This is to say, they decided to conduct a smaller ceremony than a regular *ngillatun* ritual. The ceremony was smaller both in terms of its duration and the number of people invited. Thus, it meant less effort by people who were supposed to cook for fewer guests and spend less money.

Usually, machi preside over the ceremonies of the communities in which they were born, married or bought land. In turn, communities can invest a lot of resources and time supporting the initiation process of a young person with a machi spirit. Mapuche communities that do not have a machi of their own can search for a machi in other communities. Thus, some machi preside over ceremonies in many different places. A machi who is invited to preside over ceremonies increases their reputation. Ceremonies are also an opportunity to exercise a role in the transmission of cultural practices. Thus, these are moments when machi exercise their authority beyond the medical domain. Nevertheless, these ceremonies have a preventive medical effect in at least two ways. First, they generate a sense of belonging, connectedness, and shared self-worth. Second, they provide concrete moral guidance as to how people should behave to avoid illnesses and misfortunes. In this way, preventive ritual events provide a vehicle through which machi enhance their authority and people's trust in their powers as shamans.

A *Ngillatun* Ritual in Machi Carmen's Community

The ceremony started at seven in the morning in the *ngillatuwe* (the ceremonial place). The ceremonial site was located on the property adjoining the property of the machi. The owner was one of the members of the community. Due to its ceremonial function the place was not used either for planting or for feeding the animals. The *rewe* or altar was in its center. The ceremony started by dressing the *rewe* [S: *vestir el rewe*]. The old, dry branches were removed and exchanged for fresh branches that were collected the previous day. They used branches of four native trees: *canelo* (canelo), *maqui* (Chilean wineberry), *maitén* (mayten) and *quillay* (soap bark tree). A branch of each native tree, of the same height, was placed on each side of the carved trunk and joined using strings of *coligüe* rods or ropes. Thus, the *rewe* looked like a shrub or small tree.

While several men were dressing the *rewe*, the rest of the group danced a ritual type of dancing called *pürun*. In this dance, short steps and circular movements, as well as forward and backward movements, predominate. Men and women did the same movements, but they formed columns of men alternating with columns of women. In turn, these columns formed a semicircle around the *rewe*. On other occasions, men could be seen forming various columns closer to the *rewe* and women forming columns at the back. In any case, the most important people conducting the ceremony remained in the column closest to the *rewe* where gender division of columns is less strict. Thus, the machi, headman, *zugumachife* (the person who speaks to the spirits while the machi is in trance), *llankan* (dancers who animate the machi) and other people assisting the machi remained closest to the *rewe*. The machi led the music playing her *kultrun* (ritual drum) while dancing. Machi Carmen was surrounded by four *llankan*: two women with *maqui* (Chilean wineberry) branches in their hands and two men holding *coligüe* rods with blue and white flags tied at the ends. The four *llancan* remained dancing *pürun* around the machi throughout the ceremony. The machi was also accompanied by two other women playing drums and several men playing wind instruments. Wind instruments are mostly played by men, and they consist fundamentally of *trutruka* (part of the trumpet family) and *pifüllka* (a kind of ductless flute). The monotonous rhythm was periodically interrupted by the *afafan* (shout of encouragement), which is meant to scare evil spirits and animate the audience. In addition, the sound of the *wiño* (a wooden cane used in the *palin* game or ritual hockey) hitting each other is meant to drive away evil spirits and keep the audience's mood high.

After the *rewe* was dressed, they proceeded to conduct a *llellipun* (prayer) in the form of a chant. First, the headman and older men who could speak Mapudungun rolled in front of the *rewe*. They prayed aloud, as in a lament, asking *Ngünechen* or God for the welfare and good health of the group, while the machi and other women played the *kultrun* in a low volume. Every individual participating in the prayer was saying something different. The prayer was done four times and was interrupted each time by shouts of encouragement and the loud sounds of the *kultrun* and wind instruments. After the men, the machi and other old women who could speak Mapudungun did the same as the men. The prayer was again done four times, interrupted by the *afafan* and loud music. After the first part of the ceremony, breakfast was served.

The ceremonial place was organized in *ramadas* that surrounded the site where the *rewe* was located. The *ramadas* are sheds made of branches of trees. In those places, families cook and cater to their *witran* (guests). The *ramadas* have a roof but no walls.

A little before noon, the second part of the ceremony began. This was the longest and most important, lasting about two hours. All the participants danced the *pürun* ritual dance. The machi danced and played her *kultrun*. She was the focus of attention because the audience was expecting her to go into trance. The machi was leading the participants, thus everybody was situated behind her. Only the four *llancan* (ritual dancers) danced in front and behind her, surrounding her. The sound of the ritual drum was permanent and was accompanied by the sound of wind instruments. In addition, at regular intervals, the monotony of the music was interrupted by the shout of the *afafan* (Mapuche shout of encouragement), as well as the sound of the *wiño* (wooden canes) beating each other. Also, assistants of the machi threw, on regular intervals, spring water [S: *agua de vertiente*], *mote* (boiled wheat grains) and humid leaves of medicinal plants over the heads of the participants. Everybody who was involved in the ceremony knew they were responsible for facilitating trance. This was a long and laborious process that required the participation of many people performing different roles. While participating in the ritual, it was noted how hard the work was. The participants danced for two hours, maintaining a level of expectation and tension. The expressions on their faces were of extreme concentration and physical effort. The whole group concentrated its attention on the machi, and eyes were placed on her. There was a shared expectation that the machi would go into trance and deliver an important message to the group.

Although the machi was the center of attention, the number of people needed to facilitate trance greatly exceeded just one. Thus, although the machi is the only individual experiencing trance, this could not happen without the participation of many others in different roles. In fact, before the beginning of the ceremony, Machi Carmen was worried that Bruno, the man who led the group of men playing the *pifüllka* (ductless flute), had not arrived. "I need the sound of his *pifüllka*," Machi Carmen told me. Bruno arrived when the ceremony had already begun. The way he played was louder, stronger, and more confident than the rest. Easily, one could distinguish the sound that came out of Bruno's *pifüllka*. In addition, he was the one who kept the pace, and the younger or less experienced musicians watched and followed him.

Like Bruno, other people played a fundamental role. Sonia, the wife of one of the *longko*, and Carmen's close friend, played the *kultrun* near the machi throughout the ceremony. In addition to that, she directed a small group of women who stimulated the machi by throwing humid medicinal leaves, *mote* and pumpkin seeds on her face and body. The women were permanently spitting spring water, sea water, and *muday* (an alcoholic beverage produced by the fermentation of wheat or corn grains) over the head and body of the machi, as well as over the rest of the participants. In this way, they were creating a shared sensory experience, such as the smell of the humid and fresh leaves and the touch of the water and *muday* on our faces. In addition, small pots of clay with *muday* were distributed among the participants by these women and everybody drank from them. These multisensory experiences, together with the movement of bodies following the same rhythm, created a sense of togetherness and connectedness. "Effervescence" is culturally generated by the above techniques of grasping everybody's attention through shared movement, touch, smell, and drinking. The shared expectation and attention focused on the machi and her coming trance, predisposed the participants to be actively engaged with the actions taking place and with what could happen. Thus, they are not passive receivers of the spirits' message, rather they are actively making the spirits come through their concrete actions over the machi's body. Collins

(2004: 120) claims that pride is an emotion elicited by ritual shared action. This observation coincides with observations made during my fieldwork. The people who participated in this ceremony revitalized a common feeling of self-worth, based on the value of Mapuche cultural practices and knowledge. This new sense of pride and shared self- worth contrasted with common everyday experiences of racial and class discrimination.

The changes in the conduct of a machi that allow one to know that they are in a trance are, in general, subtle. The machi dances with their eyes closed, the dance becomes more energetic, they eat *canelo* leaves. Sometimes, changes in conduct are more dramatic, such as undressing, running great distances, jumping into rivers or streams, or dangerously throwing knives in the air. Because of their previous experiences with the ceremony, people were expectant about what was going to happen to the machi this time and what they were going to say. In the event I am describing, Machi Carmen danced more energetically and with her eyes closed. She also started avidly eating *canelo* leaves, which protect her against evil spirits. In this state, she climbed the steps of the *rewe* to stand at the tip. There she waved the branches of the *rewe* energetically. The participants cheered her with shouts and music. The *zugumachife* now acquired a significant role. He silenced the participants so that the spirit of the machi could speak. The spirit came waving: "*Mari mari pu peñi*" (good day brothers), "*Mari mari pu lamgnen*" (good day sisters).[12] The audience responded, "*Mari, mari*" (good day). The message was delivered in the form of a chant accompanied by the *kultrun* in a low tone and a slow pace. The machi periodically played her *kultrun* faster and louder, which was a signal for the participants to play their instruments and shout cries of encouragement. Then, people were silent again, so the spirit could proceed to speak. The *zungumachife* helped the audience to know when to encourage the spirit and when to remain silent. The *zugumachife* replied to the spirit while the machi was in trance. He or she can ask questions, explain problems and worries, and encourage, greet, or thank the machi spirit.

Ritual chants and prayers during trance follow a predetermined script to some extent. First, the spirit greeted the audience and said it was coming as a *werken* (messenger) because the machi requested its presence. The spirits usually tell the audience their trajectory to get there. Then, the spirit gave information about the *wallmapu* (universe), to then refer to closer places. Finally, the spirit gave information about individuals or families. The language spoken during trance is Mapudungun, though certain words are also borrowed from Spanish. On this occasion, the spirit said the machi was sad because she was alone (she had recently become a widow). In addition, the spirit reprimanded the *longko* (headman), who forgot to pick up the machi at her house before the beginning of the ceremony, as befits the ritual protocol. Also, the spirit announced coming natural events. They were going to experience a tremor soon. They should not be scared but go to the ocean and pray for protection. The spirit calmed those present, telling them that because they have performed the ceremony they were going to be safe from natural disasters.

The machi's trance coincides with what Turner (1977) described as the liminal phase of ritual. The status of liminal individuals is socially and structurally ambiguous. The kind of social group emerging in a liminal moment is an unstructured or rudimentarily structured and relatively undifferentiated communion of equal individuals who submit together to the authority of the ritual leaders. In this way, ritual revitalizes social structure (ibid.), while making individuals part of its normative dimension. At the same time, ritual allows for renegotiations of social conflicts, as well as new productions of meaning. In this case, the spirits' message reaffirms the moral necessity of the continuity of Mapuche cultural practices. The message delivered during trance points to the moral obligation the group has in maintaining the Mapuche lifeworld (to continue to perform the *ngillatun* ritual). If the group fulfills this obligation, the universe will maintain its balance, preventing the occurrence of natural disasters and misfortunes. The need for survival of the Mapuche practices appears in a context in which people feel the continuity of their existence as a group threatened.

After delivering the message, the machi descended from the *rewe* and continued to dance and play her ritual drum. The dance continued for approximately thirty more minutes. After trance, the tension was reduced, so people danced in a more relaxed and cheerful way. The machi, still in trance, periodically started to run aimlessly with all the crowd following her. People ran after the machi laughing, in a joyful mood. Joy and contagious energy have been described as vehicles for revitalizing social structures and norms (e.g., Kapferer

1991; Plancke 2014). Running behind the machi in trance was understood by those present as an activity to protect her from an imprudent action. As the machi was still in a trance, her conduct was erratic. The way the group ran behind her to prevent her from leaving the *ngillatuwe* (ceremonial site) was joyful and playful. You could hear laughter and expressions such as "grab her," "do not let her go." Nobody really grabbed her, rather people surrounded her, constraining her movements. On the other hand, the machi found the space between the participants to manage to run away from the group for a few seconds, until she was again surrounded. Finally, the *zungumachife* and the male *llancan* energetically wiped two *wiños* (wooden cane used in the *palin* game) on the body of the machi from head to toe, while she was surrounded by the female *llancan* and other close people. By this action they were making the spirit leave the machi's body.

The closing of the ceremony is a conversation around the *rewe*. The machi, the headman and other old men and women sat in the first column closest to the *rewe*. The *zugumachife* repeated to the machi and the rest of the audience what the spirit said while she was in trance (a machi in trance is possessed, so she does not remember anything that happened). This provided an opportunity to reflexively construct meaning and solve social conflicts. The headman acknowledged that he had made a mistake when he did not go to pick up the machi at her home. In addition, the recent widowhood of the machi and her feelings of loneliness are acknowledged by the group. Also, this part of the ceremony is an opportunity for any participant to raise an issue of concern. In this event, a Mapuche community from Argentina took the opportunity to share concerns about how to hold their own ceremony. They explained to the audience that the reason for their visit was to learn from them because they were having many doubts about how to perform their own traditional ceremonies. Some people discussed formal aspects of the ceremony that could have been done better. For example, an old woman reprimanded people who stayed in the *ramadas* cooking, eating, or chatting instead of participating in the ceremony. Moreover, some young people asked for the spirits' message to be translated. Most young people do not speak Mapudungun. The *longko* agreed, but at the same time he used the opportunity to try to convince young people to learn Mapudungun.

After the discussion, the participants performed a festive and playful dance called *choike pürun* (ostrich dance). Four men danced, imitating the ostrich mating dance while inviting women to dance with them. Men fought between each other for the women as male ostriches do. The rivalry for women generated laughter in the audience. Some people accompanied the dancers playing instruments or simply watched. Others commented on who was the best dancer. The most flirtatious and bold dancers were the ones people liked the most. "*Ese choike sí que es gallo* (that ostrich is indeed a rooster)," I heard a man saying. After the *choike pürun*, people had lunch. People sat in the *ramadas* of the families they belonged to or the families that invited them. I sat with the machi and her family and friends. Food was served in abundance. People took home large quantities of food, mostly cow and pork meat, in plastic bags. Women cooked but men served their guests. Men went *ramada* by *ramada* serving food to other families in their community and the guests of those other families. Lunchtime was long and enjoyable, and people remained eating and chatting until five or six in the afternoon.

A key element of ritual is crafting a performative order through repetition, creating a subjunctive world in which boundaries are negotiated and relations are redefined (Seligman et al. 2008: 17–42). The aim is to participate in shared action to create a shared physical and emotional experience, and a sense of community. Bodies fall into shared rhythms, and a sense of unity arises. An important factor behind the creation of a sense of community among performers is the link with previous performers. People remarked that they were doing what their ancestors did, in the same way and place their ancestors performed. The alerting quality (Lewis 1980) of ritual seeks to achieve shared experience through the creation of shared sensorial experience (Hsu 2005, 2008). Furthermore, ritual action aims to achieve a shared emotional experience of, first, anxiety and expectation, and then relief through laughter and joy.

A real machi, then, plays a fundamental role in the creation of a sense of togetherness. By presiding over ceremonies, they become indispensable for the continuity of the group. Thus, they gain legitimacy as a real machi due to their role in building community. She/he is not the only social actor indispensable for community building. Importantly, they need many different people performing different roles to perform a successful ceremony. In this way, a large number of community members can have an active and significant role in a ceremony, generating a shared sense of self-worth.

In summary, I have discussed how machi divine, treat, and generate trust in their powers and diminish the ambiguity of them. To do so, machi engage in divinatory techniques that allow them to construct a problem and prescribe a solution. These techniques seek to promote imagination through the direction of attention and induction of negative affective states. Together with their role in divining and treating aliments and misfortunes, machi play a role in community building. By presiding over group ceremonies, machi become indispensable in revitalizing social practices and solving social conflicts.

Notes

1. For issues of clarity, I use the word patient. However, the term is too narrow to describe the various types of relationships machi have with the people they treat. There are other words that are used more frequently, such as son (S: *hijo*) or daughter (S: *hija*) to refer to young people; mummy (S: *mamita*) to refer in an affectionate way to another woman; *papai* to refer in an affectionate but solemn way to an old woman or to a woman whom one admires and respect; *chachai* to refer in an affectionate but solemn way to an old man or a man worthy of respect and admiration. Machi and patients are usually close friends or even relatives who refer to each other by their names. When a machi does not want to mention the name of a person they treated, she or he is usually referred to as "the sick person" (S: *el enfermo/a*). No machi I knew would use the word client due to the instrumental connotation of the term.
2. This observation has also been described by other ethnographers working with Mapuche shamans (e.g., Bacigalupo 2001, 2007).
3. Conversion rates are those of 2018.
4. Minimum wage in 2017.
5. The word *rewe* can also refer to the altar in the center of a *ngillatun* ritual site, the place in which a *ngillatun* ritual takes place, and to a ritual congregation (Course 2011: 140). In the case of machi, once they install a *rewe* in a place, they locate their machi's spirit in that place. Thus, a machi must maintain permanent physical contact with their *rewe*, as well as provide permanent care to it. If a machi moves from a place, for example, if they marry, they should take their *rewe* with them.
6. In Spanish, people used to say *ver la orina* (see the urine). People used the verb "to see" instead of "to look" (S: *mirar*). "To see" refers to the capacity for vision, whereas "to look" refers to focusing attention on specific things we see. Thus, my interlocutors were referring to a specific capacity for

seeing; that is, to see the urine is something that only a machi or a person with a spiritual gift can do.

7. University enrolment has grown exponentially in Chile since the 1990s. Many students are the first generation of their family going to university, and this is also the case among the Mapuche. The expansion of undergraduate programs was not accompanied by adequate regulation. In this way, many undergraduate programs were closed due to the lack of any work market for graduates they produced, as well as legal irregularities (and bankruptcy) within higher education institutions. In this case, the woman was going to end up with a university diploma of a program that was going to cease to exist. For this reason, her university education will have little value when looking for better paid jobs (due to the diminished reputation of the program in which she studied). In the Chilean context, her frustration and anxiety about the future are immediately understood without further explanation, because what she is experiencing is a common situation.
8. This refers to the audible sounds the guts produce while moving. It could be painful but most commonly it is not.
9. For a summary of the first chronicles about the *ngillatun* ritual see Zapater (1998). For more recent accounts, see Bacigalupo (2007: 64–72) and Course (2011: 138–59).
10. My interlocutors also used the word ceremony to refer to other rituals such as healing rituals.
11. The construction of hydroelectric power plants has produced devastating social, economic, and environmental consequences. Its opposition is one significant trigger of a strong indigenous movement in Chile (see Baquedano 2004 for an account of the emblematic Ralco case).
12. It is common for a female machi to be possessed by a male spirit, as was the case in the event described here. It is possible to know the spirit is masculine due to the way he speaks. *Peñi* (brother) is a word that only men use when referring to other men. Instead, women use the word *lamgen* (brother or sister) to refer to both women and men. See Bacigalupo (2007: 87–90) for an account on the gendered relations between machi and their spirits.

Chapter 3
Techniques for Seeing the Evil Spirit

In the previous chapter, I described how a machi can see illnesses and misfortunes through *pewtun* techniques. Here, I discuss the communal seeing of evil spirits (Mapudungun: *wekufe, wezanewen*; Spanish: *demonio, espíritu malo*) in the context of ritual healing. While the machi is the one seeing in the case of *pewtun* techniques, here all ritual participants should see. Seeing constitutes a mode of self-process (Csordas 1994a) through which people experience a sensorial and affective shift. This shift is one from a sense of loss of control to demonic/external/chaotic influences, to a sense of release from unwanted intrusions and regaining self-control.

Seeing the evil spirit is an imaginative act involving multisensory modalities and negative affective states, such as fear. Images of an evil spirit are ritually induced to produce moments of synchronicity (Hsu 2005) or, as I call them here, moments of communal seeing. Through communal seeing, an active and creative engagement with a situation is promoted. Moreover, as seeing is an act shared by a group of participants, a sense of acting together against an evil force is produced. The communal seeing of evil spirits, through active sensory and affective engagement, is essential to ritual performative efficacy. Ritual action is firstly directed at objectifying and localizing the evil spirit and then expelling and disposing of it.

Different sensory modalities allow people to see evil spirits: visual images, auditory images, haptic images, and negative emotions, such as fear. However, visual images are the predominant sensory modality. The fact that vision is the preferred sensory modality is evident in what I will describe below regarding a machi's inculcation of visual imagery. Many of my informants emphasized the fact that biomedical diagnostic techniques cannot visualize the negative effects of evil spirits on people's bodies. Therefore, machi are thought to be the only type of practitioners that can make evil spirits visible. Images of evil spirits are experienced as sudden, involuntary and embodied, and they are non-symbolically linked to evil spirits due to contiguity; that is, they are indexes with varying degrees of iconicity. Put another way, they are immediately understood as the presence of an evil force without the necessity of further explanation or conceptual analyses. Frequently, images of evil spirits are indications of the pragmatics of an ongoing ritual healing event (Csordas 1994a: 96): they are intuitively understood as the confirmation that an evil spirit is indeed causing the affliction, and as an indication that evil spirits are vulnerable to healing action.

Evil Spirits and Witchcraft in the Mapuche Context

The healing practices described in this chapter are different to the practices described in Chapter 2 in several respects. *Pewtun* and *ngillatun* rituals (as well as the *zatun* ritual described in Chapter 4) are considered "authentic" expressions of tradition and spirituality by Mapuche people and state authorities. *Pewtun* ritual is officially sponsored by the state since it occurs within state-financed institutions. Some Mapuche communities invite state authorities, such as mayors or members of CONADI (National Corporation of Indigenous Issues), to participate in their *ngillatun* ritual.[1] In addition, children learn at school detailed descriptions about the *ngillatun* and other Mapuche traditional ceremonies, and they must answer exam questions about them. In contrast, the ritual actions described in this chapter are more idiosyncratic to individual machi and are kept within the domestic realm (participating individuals are kin or close friends). Thus, these events belong to a private sphere and are endowed with secrecy. Moreover, in the ritual events described here, evil spirits have a predominant role both as explanatory causes of illness and misfortune, as well as a target of ritual action. In the first event described, that of the ritual search of the *entierro* (buried object), witchcraft is the source of illness and conflict. In the second event, that of the *ulutun* ritual,[2] the negative effects of evil spirits on a person's health are the result of unintended consequences. Significantly, while rituals described in Chapter 2 (as well as those described in Chapters 4 and 5) could be understood, at least in part, as part of a revivalist movement and struggles for identity, the events presented here do not primarily seek to affirm a Mapuche identity nor to enroll people into collective ritual life. Rather, the healing actions discussed in this chapter are directed toward occult forces that endanger people's lives and wellbeing. Not surprisingly, I observe that this type of healing is as popular among Mapuche as it is among non-Mapuche.

Illness, death, and personal crises are frequently considered to be the result of the evil intentions of other people or of human reckless behavior and negative emotions, such as anger or envy. People have the power to do evil because they can deliberately manipulate or non-willfully mobilize evil spirits. Evil spirits can destroy the integrity of a person and subjugate their will. However, for the evil spirit to have a negative effect on a person, they must be weak. The weakness (S: *debilidad*) that makes people vulnerable to witchcraft and evil spirits originates in personal *yafkan* (moral transgressions) whether deliberate or not, that disrupt a web of relations between the person and their world. These transgressions are commonly related to the betrayal of the Mapuche way of *küme mognen* (good living). Actions (or omissions) constituting such a betrayal could be the following: not participating in the *ngillatun* ritual; neglecting to teach the children to speak Mapudungun; neglecting spiritual and leadership duties when it comes to machi or headmen; or using a ceremonial site as an area for cultivating the land. Individuals, families or communities may have committed transgressions. In addition, they could have been committed in the past but affect members of a family or community in the present. "Many of the diseases come from an ethical transgression, they may even have been a transgression of a grandparent or of a parent," a friend told me. Thus, the victim is frequently considered to be responsible for their own misfortune and their own recovery.

Some of the cases in which evil spirits are considered the cause of diseases are clearly cases of witchcraft (M: *kalkutun*; S: *brujería*); that is, a person is deliberately trying to hurt another person through the manipulation of evil spirits. When people think this is the case, they usually say, "An evil was done to me" (S: *me hicieron un daño*). While conducting fieldwork in the 1990s, Bacigalupo (2001: 55) observed that witchcraft (M: *kalkutun*) was the most frequent disease machi treated. I observed that, although witchcraft remains a common way of explaining illnesses and misfortunes, other more ambiguous and complex explanations about the involvement of evil spirits in people's suffering were as common as witchcraft among Mapuche people (but less so among non-Mapuche people). People refer to ailments and misfortunes caused by evil spirits as *wezakutran* (an illness caused by an evil spirit). Witchcraft may or may not be the cause of *wezakutran*.

While trying to hurt another person through witchcraft is considered unambiguously morally reproachable, the involvement of evil spirits as agents of sickness is morally ambiguous. For instance, some people thought that spirits could not be considered evil, as they were just trying to catch the attention of people who had forgotten about their ancestors and traditional ways of living: "If someone overexploits the land, leaving it unsuited for further agricultural work, or if someone cuts down native trees, the *ngen* [spiritual guardians] of such places and beings bring spiritual diseases upon people to call their attention, to show what they are doing wrong," a friend told me. For some of my interlocutors, to blame the spirits (or witches) was a way of avoiding responsibility. Moreover, the spirits' bringing of illness and misfortune could be understood as a warning sign that, if understood and dealt with properly, could help to restore balance and health. In this way, some of my informants said that the spirits were helping people. Also, when magic is used to obtain personal benefits, such as keeping the beloved person tied to a loving bond, and not to harm another person, it can be morally acceptable. For example, a machi told me that she uses love magic to protect a marriage tie but not to help a woman attract an already married man. In this way, although my informants frequently talked about evil (S: *mal* or *maldad*) as a source of suffering and illness, the moral ramifications are multiple and ambiguous, rather than only perverse and diabolic. This is in line with what Parkin (1985) already noted about descriptions of evil in *The Anthropology of Evil*:

> It can refer to extreme fear, death and destruction, but also to lesser misfortunes. It may denote an agent's firm intention to harm, or instead may be seen as originating in an unintended human or non-human condition. Evil agents may be abhorrent, but they may also be admired for their cleverness. While people may be terrified of the deadly effects of the worst

> kinds of evil, they can at other times joke about it and make humorous parallel. Talk about evil thus ranges over the terrible and serious as well as the playful and creative.
>
> (Parkin 1985: 1)

In this chapter, I describe two ritual healing events in which machi dealt successfully with evil spirits. This is to say that the evil spirits were identified, expelled, and disposed of through ritual action. The first event, that of searching for the *entierro* (buried object), corresponds to a case of witchcraft. Here, a person deliberately wanted to hurt a family by burying an object attached to an evil spirit in their courtyard. The buried object needed to be found and disposed of to treat the negative effects it was having on all members of a family. In the second event, that of Rosa and her family, evil spirits had attacked the patient both because she was weak (due to a medical disease) and because of the irresponsibility of a machi. Therefore, the harmful effects of evil spirits on a person's body were the result of both personal vulnerabilities and human reckless behavior. What is similar in both cases is the insistence of the machi that people should see the evil spirit. Only after seeing the evil spirit is it possible to proceed to expel it so that people can get rid of evil influences in their lives. "If you don't see it [the evil spirit], it will stay with you," I was warned by a machi. In other words, after the evil spirit is visualized, proper ritual action can be directed against it. Therefore, machi promote the seeing of evil spirits through different ritual techniques.

Searching for the *Entierro*

In what follows, I discuss a ritual healing occasion in which a Mapuche family, with the help of a machi, searches and finds a buried object attached to an evil spirit that was left in their courtyard by a witch. The heads of the family were an older couple, in their fifties, who were originally from an Indigenous community close to Temuco and migrated to a city further south due to economic hardship. The couple lived with their children and a grandchild, and I will refer to them as mother and father. The father earned a small salary for a job in a custom office. His salary was complemented by the family business run by the mother. They lived in a big, old, wooden house of three floors and about ten rooms, where they hosted several lodgers who paid for a room to sleep and some meals. In addition, they had clients who rented improvised makeshift rooms that had been recently built in the courtyard of the house. This business was an informal one and their clients were mostly men who had come from other areas of the country seeking seasonal jobs. The mother also worked as a machi and received patients in her house. Their economic situation was above the poverty line, but they depended on credit and were indebted. Revenue from their business varied significantly so the only stable income they had was the father's salary. Sometimes they struggled to pay the bills and the rent, the machi told me. However, they had managed to buy a car and a taxi license for their son, who was working as an independent taxi driver. The couple's son lived with his parents together with his partner and their toddler son. The older couple also had a teenage daughter who, during the ritual event, was sleeping and, like the toddler, did not participate in the ritual. Thus, the participating individuals were the mother, the father, the son and his partner, together with the machi and me. I will refer to the individuals in this way since the problem was a family issue rather than only a condition of one individual.

The family had known the machi for several years. They had come to know her because friends had recommended the machi as a good healer. Although the family was originally from a rural area close to the Indigenous community of origin of the machi, they had met her through friends and acquaintances in the city. Usually, when people consider a machi has treated them effectively they will turn to them again every time they face illnesses or crises. They will also bring their family members and friends to the machi in case of need. Therefore, a machi becomes an important person to all members of a family or a network of kin and friends.

The machi and I arrived after midnight following a four-hour car journey. It was dark, cold and wet due to heavy rain during the day. The son had picked us up from the house of the machi. Upon arrival, the women of the family rushed to serve us food. I was struck by the prevailing silence. The women silently and laboriously hurried to serve the food while the men sat with the machi and me at the kitchen table. Except for the routine question about the health of the machi and her family, we sat and ate in silence. The men seemed tense: the son sighed loudly and repeatedly, the father clumsily tried to help his wife and daughter-in-law to serve the food. The father asked the women to hurry, and the mother responded in an irritated tone for him to stop bothering her.

After eating, and with all the participants seated at the kitchen table, the machi suddenly asked for a glass of water. This request interrupted the silence. The mother handed the machi a glass of water, and she put it on the kitchen table and stared at it closely. The machi's actions were closely followed by all the participants, who had their eyes on her. Nobody said anything, and I noted that people were hardly moving at all. The participants were staring at the machi in a state of tense motionless. In this way, the machi's action of carefully staring at the glass of water was immediately followed by an attentive and tense silence. To focus everybody's attention on the glass of water is a technique generating synchronicity (Hsu 2005). In this way, all the participants are grasped by the same existential and sensorial experience: looking at the glass of water. The technical production of synchronicity allows for a shared somatic experience and engages the participants in the situation.

The moment of synchronicity described above increased the tension. The son was the most expressive individual: I could hear his sighs becoming louder and more frequent. He suddenly leaned back, away from the table, and grabbed his head. His mother touched him on the shoulder, gently causing him to move toward the table again. The mother said: "We need to be calm and stay together."

Together with increasing the tension, synchronicity is an indication that action will take place, that something is going to happen. Thus, it promoted active engagement and led to a discussion in which the family verbalized (the mother had the leading voice, but all the members contributed to the discussion) what was wrong with them and explored possible explanations. They were continuously arguing with each other and the couples living in the house did not seem to get along. The father was especially irritable and reacted aggressively to common family discussions and disagreements. In addition, they were all sleeping poorly because they were hearing creaks all over the house at night. The teenage daughter of the older couple had a rash on her skin that was itching significantly and was also very distant from the rest of the family, always locked up in her room, appearing sad and fatigued. The son was not able to earn enough money to be economically independent because the taxi that he drove was constantly breaking down. He had spent a lot of money repairing the car. They believed all these misfortunes, symptoms, and disagreements between them were happening due to the act of one evil person and her accomplices. Somebody had left an *entierro* (buried object), which usually contains earth from a cemetery, bones of death animals, and maybe human or animal hair, among multiple other possibilities. With the *entierro*, an evil spirit was positioned in the family's home and was having negative physical and psychological consequences on people and their relations. Thus, the buried object is the "materialization," as they explained to me, of a spirit or energy manipulated by an evil person to hurt another person or a family. The evil one or the "traitor" can do it alone or with the help of a witch. It is a serious threat and can lead to death if proper measures are not taken. They seemed to know who the person who wished them wrong was. The evil one was the ex-partner of the son, who had lived with the family for a couple of years and could never overcome the anger after the son decided to break up with her. As the son had recently had a baby with his new partner, the jealousy and envy had intensified. Although they knew the identity of the one responsible, they were more interested in knowing who the mediator was; that is, the person who had left the buried object in the house and the one who fabricated it. Moreover, although they knew the son's ex-partner had used black magic against them in the past, they did not have any proof to blame her this time. Therefore, it was possible that other people were involved. The mother worried about other machi who might be jealous of her success in treating patients in the city. "Do you think one of our lodgers may be the one?" the mother asked the machi. The machi replied that nobody would pay rent to do black magic, it would be too expensive. The machi then added that she had told them to put cameras in the house. The family acknowledged she had advised them to do so but went on to explain various practical reasons why it was difficult to do so, including the price. The advice about installing cameras made it obvious that this had happened before. I will come back to the chronicity of this case below.

The conversation above contains multiple concerns, explanations, and questions about possible courses of action that remain open and incomplete. Should they take their teenage daughter to the doctor? What can the son do to earn more money? Can they trust their lodgers? Could they catch the witch with cameras? Multiple worries, explanations, and courses of action are discussed in a disorganized way, which increases the dramatic tension of the moment. Problems and doubts about what action to take seem to build up instead of being clarified or ordered. Parkin (1991) used the term "cognitive simultaneity" when describing the multiple, divergent, and even chaotic possibilities of explanation of a diviner's speech. Whyte (1997: 67–70) described the same technique used by diviners in eastern Uganda and referred to it as "the construction of uncertainty."[3] According to Whyte, diviners need first to perform uncertainty to later perform order and certainty through ritual action. When clients go to diviners to ask who the witch is, uncertainty is built up in a deliberate way.

> [B]oth client and diviner should begin a seance in a state of uncertainty. This uncertainty is not simply "there." It is constructed and emphasized. The declarations of ignorance and confusion are artificial in a sense: the client might well have his suspicion, and the diviner's uncertainty is imposed by the convention that he or she should not ask directly for the facts of the case.
>
> (Whyte 1997: 68)

Abruptly interrupting the discussion about who had left the *entierro* and whether cameras were a feasible method to catch the witch, the machi asked for a fork to be put inside the glass of water. Then, she kept staring at the glass closely. This again generated a tense silence. Suddenly, she put the glass in front of the son and asked him, "What do you see?" The son was hesitant and did not reply. The machi added firmly, "Everybody needs to see it, otherwise it may stay with you." The machi initially gave some suggestions as to what could be seen in the glass of water with a fork in it: "The fork has six prongs instead of five," she said. This is a vague image that is more an invitation to see and engage with the situation than a sign to be interpreted. Gradually, words came out from different people to describe what they were seeing in that glass full of water with a fork in it, while it was passing from hand to hand: "A woman's face, her hair, a dog, a cat … it appears and disappears."[4] The shared images were not attempted to be put together into a coherent system of meaning, rather their appearance intensified the feelings of fear toward something invisible and vague. What is important is to see it. In this context, the images are indexically linked to the object (i.e., the evil spirit). There is no necessity to conceptually explain what the images mean because people share an immediate and intuitive understanding that these images are the "materialization," as they say, of an evil spirit.

The vision of evil spirits acts as an objectifying mechanism: the evil spirit, in this way, loses its intrusive effect and people can search for it, find it, and expel it from their home and body. My observations are like those of Stroeken (2008), who contrasted the objectifying and detaching seeing of healers, as opposed to the intrusive seeing of witches, in the case of the Sukuma. "Victims call the witch (*nogi*) emphatically *ngwi-bon-eeji*, literally, 'the one who persistently makes you see yourself'" (ibid.: 476). Therefore, witchcraft supposes an intrusive seer or witch who stares in a way that kills. Divination through the inspection of the entrails and feathers of sacrificed birds identifies the witch through visible marks interpreted by the healer. The treatment of witchcraft in the event described here, as in the Sukuma case, depends on forms of exteriorizing through objectifying and detaching sensorial experiences. In this way, it is possible to confirm that an evil spirit is in fact the agent causing the affliction and that it is now pertinent to initiate ritual actions against it.

The ritual proceeded by the machi asking the son to tell us where he thought the *entierro* was. The previously doubtful, hesitant, and fearful participant replied immediately. He told us that one night he heard creaking in one of the corners of the room where he slept with his partner. He decided to follow those creaks, which went down the outer wall into the courtyard of the house. In the yard, he stopped at the last place where he heard the creaks and began to dig. He wanted to find the buried object and destroy it. While he was doing this, "a dog came out of nowhere" and attacked him. He was so scared that he stopped digging and decided not to continue to seek the buried object alone. He realized he needed the help of a machi because the "bad energy" deposited there was too powerful. The image of an unprovoked aggressive dog was immediately understood as the materialization of an evil force, without any further explanation. What is intuitively evil about this image is not the dog but the unprovoked aggression of a commonly unaggressive animal (street dogs in Chile are not aggressive). The machi asked him to bring dust from the very same spot he tried to dig at. He did as the machi told him and added the dust to the glass full of water with a fork in it. "Now you can see it clearly," said the machi.

After "seeing it clearly," we started preparing for the actual search for the *entierro*. In this way, the objectification of the evil spirit through the sense of vision allows the transition to the second part of the ritual treatment: the search for the *entierro*. A buried object attached to an evil spirit through black magic must be found and thrown into a river or a moving body of water. The preparation for the search consisted of putting herbs that are counterhexes (S: *contras*), such as rue, inside pockets and clothes. One important characteristic of counterhex plants and herbs is that they are aromatic herbs. In addition, an incense burner (S: *sahumerio*) was prepared, which contained garlic, chili pepper and other counterhexes. We also spat *aguardiente* (a grape distillate with high alcohol content) at the house's backyard door, before going out to the courtyard. *Aguardiente* is also a substance with a strong smell and taste. The machi spoke in Mapudungun to the spirit, commanding it to leave the house: "The evil person who sent you and left you here as the guardian of this *entierro* is trying to hurt this family, so I come, as a machi, to pay you to go, because I need to take what you are protecting." The counterhexes are used to overcome the resistance of the evil spirit, so it can finally leave and the *entierro* can be found and disposed of.

After protecting our bodies using counterhexes and weakening the evil spirit through seeing it, we went to the place where the dog had appeared while the son was digging. It was dark, so the father was lighting the way with a flashlight. The machi pinned her knife in the place where the son had tried to dig and then ordered the son to "feel it," to "grab the knife and feel it." The son grabbed the knife and immediately felt an electric current running through his body, which scared him and caused him to release the knife. Contrary to visual images of the evil spirit, a haptic image had a negative effect on the ritual search. The intense fear caused by the sensation of electricity inside the body caused the son to become weak and unable to continue with the search. After this event, the machi became the sole protagonist of the search. This confirmed the family's perception that the evil spirit was so powerful that only a machi could find it and expel it.

Immediately after the son released the knife, the machi shouted: "Do not let go!" The machi grabbed the knife pinned in the ground and said: "I see it, it is moving, there it is! Everybody has to see it, so it will not stay with you." We all saw a blue-white light moving around the knife pinned to the ground. *Aguardiente* was abundantly spilled over the spot. Then, the machi proceeded to draw dust with a shovel from around where the knife was pinned and put the dust into an empty sack of potatoes. She tied the sack, hit it hard against the ground and, again, indicated to the group how the "energy" moved inside, while we all saw the folds of the sack move. After hitting it hard enough and throwing more *aguardiente* on it, the machi opened the sack and started to search for the *entierro* in it. That moment constituted one of great tension, a climax, after a terrifying search under light rain and bitter cold. The machi finally grabbed the *entierro*, which was a pile of clothing stained with car oil, wrapped around a tarot card portraying a naked woman. Suddenly, the son's partner shouted that they had seen it before and thought it was just toilet paper. The machi was shocked to hear that, and we could all hear a small frightened sigh that emerged from her mouth.

While the sense of vision predominates in the first part of the ritual treatment, the second part is significantly more multisensory. Other sensory modalities such as the aroma of herbs and incense, as well as the strong alcoholic taste and smell of the *aguardiente*, protect the body of the participants from the lethal effects of an evil spirit. These sensory experiences serve as a harness, preparing the body for a dangerous search. The chanting voice of the machi commanding the evil spirit to leave had a similar effect. In addition, the bodies of the participants kept in contact with each other. Thus, a single body was formed, protected from the action of evil spirits.

After finding the *entierro*, the tension was reduced, and a sense of relief was evident. The search had been successful, and everybody felt that the danger of the situation was under control. The buried object found was taken by the mother, the father, the son, and the machi to the closest river and thrown into it. While they drove to do that, I stayed in the house having a conversation with the son's partner. She told me that the machi had come about three times a year to search for an *entierro* for the past three or four years. These events had started to happen long before she began living with her partner's family. She also explained that the family had recently moved from a house so that witches could not find them. All their efforts had been fruitless, and I was astonished to find out about the chronicity of the problems and the multiple episodes that had occurred. I asked whether the family had ever confronted the evil person. The young woman told me that she was told the family once confronted a male machi, a *kalku* (witch), who admitted he did black magic in exchange for money. She had not been present when that confrontation occurred. About the person who was primarily responsible, the son's ex-partner, she did not know much. She had never seen her, and the family had not seen her in years. They did not know where she lived.

Although the ritual healing act of searching for, finding, and throwing an *entierro* into a river generated a sense of self-efficacy and that a problem had been detected and solved, the chronicity of the problem seemed troublesome. Although the ritual was performatively efficacious in the sense that the evil spirit was expelled, therapeutic efficacy, understood as alleviating suffering and interpersonal conflict, was more elusive.[5]

When I told my informants about this family that was constantly being attacked by witches, they all agreed on one issue: the factor that can explain, at least in part, the chronicity of the problem is that the machi avoided confrontations with the family about their own responsibility for their repeated misfortunes. As was stated above, evil spirits can only harm people who are weak. In turn, being weak is usually related to moral transgressions. Therefore, the victim and the *ngen kutran* (victim's family) are responsible for their own misfortune due to their own personal failures.[6] A frequent transgression committed by victims of witchcraft is to have themselves participated in witchcraft practices. In fact, I later found out that the man who usually assisted the machi in these rituals refused to accompany her this time. I had a conversation with him in which he explained that he thought the mother of the family was a witch. Because the mother was a machi, it was not surprising that, among the family members, she was the suspected witch. For him, to be the continuous victim of witchcraft could only indicate that you yourself are a witch. Therefore, he did not trust the family, nor did he want his machi to maintain her long-term involvement with them. He was worried that eventually the family was going to accuse his machi of witchcraft.

The machi did not disagree with her *keyu*'s (assistant) concerns. Nevertheless, she considered that these concerns did not contradict the fact that the family was in fact being attacked by a witch.

The machi was worried about two issues. First, the witch was smart and tricky, and thus difficult to neutralize. This concern of course affirmed the importance of her role as a powerful healer. Secondly, the family did not want to talk about their own responsibility in causing their problems. When I asked her why she did not confront them, she replied that she knew they were not going to listen.

The same machi had the same concerns when dealing with another similar, although less chronic, case. This other case involved a non-Mapuche young married couple who lived in a small town even further south. They were the prosperous owners of a small business that, together with family enmities, provoked the envy of all. When I went there with the machi to search for an *entierro,* it was the second time the machi had been called for. After we found the *entierro*, I had a dream of a Mapuche community who decided to sacrifice a horse. They did it in a painful and uncompassionate way, cutting all four legs off the animal and letting it die bleeding. In my dream, I was watching the animal bleeding to death, in great pain, and I was so hurt by the image that I desperately tried to convince the headman and the elders to kill the suffering horse quickly, instead of letting it suffer. They ignored me. Then, I saw the machi, and I ran toward her to beg her to convince the headman and the elders to kill the horse rapidly. She looked at me with an expression of powerlessness and moved her arms and shoulders in a gesture of defeat. I understood she was telling me that there was nothing she could do about it. I told this dream to the machi because it is one's duty to do so. Dreams contain social and spiritual information and they must be shared. In addition, talking about the dream was an opportunity to question the machi about the effectiveness of her healing. The machi listened carefully and said that she felt exactly as I saw her in my dream. She admitted she was helpless because people in the town were going to continue to envy this family. All she could do was to provide relief to the family for a while. She did not think she could solve the interpersonal problems at the origin of the suffering the family was experiencing.

The question, then, was why she kept treating these cases if she knew she could not help. She replied, insisting on the destructive power of the evil forces she was neutralizing and, thus, evidencing her value as a healer. Nevertheless, the moral implications of her actions remained problematic, as becomes evident when listening to the reasons people gave to distrust machi. The main reasons my informants told me machi should not be trusted are the following: using tricks, accusing innocent people of witchcraft (and, thus, turning family members, friends and neighbors against each other), engaging in love magic, and even making up stories about evil spirits and witchcraft just for their own economic gain. Therefore, some machi refrain from engaging in tricks, love magic, and explicit accusations/divinations of witchcraft. Rather, they allude more abstractly to the role of spirits in calling upon individuals (through illness and misfortune) who have abandoned Mapuche ritual life or Mapuche norms and ways of living (or who have committed other forms of moral transgressions). In this way, the ritual described here is a good example of the type of activity some machi may restrain themselves from engaging in. This is a clandestine activity in which a machi can easily be suspected of bringing the *entierro* themself and, thus, cheating, purely for their own economic gain. Why does a machi get involved in these practices despite the danger they entail? Beyond the obvious reason, which is receiving money (in the event of searching for the *entierro* the machi was paid about US$150 and I found out they still owed her money from previous services), there may be other reasons related to the power that an individual obtains when dealing with occult forces. Otherwise, it would be hard to explain why machi who are prestigious and who could easily earn money in other, less ambiguous, ways, continue to participate in the search for buried objects and witches.

Machi are marginalized individuals within the dominant Chilean society; that is, they are usually portrayed as illiterate, women, backward, poor rural peasants. Machi are also usually considered to be mentally unstable, highly suggestable, and possibly dangerous to gullible individuals. Within the Mapuche society, machi are usually women who, in turn, are subjugated to men's authority. Dealing with witchcraft is a clandestine and dangerous activity that, nevertheless, can subvert an individual's marginalized position. Therefore, dealing with evil spirits can be understood as a political strategy of socially marginalized people of using their own marginality as a source of power, money, and control. Jackson (2012: 93–112) describes the same subverting strategy in the case of shape-shifting among the Kuranko of Sierra Leone. When discussing the confession of one of his informants, Mohammed, that he can shape-shift into an elephant (which is considered a form of witchcraft), Jackson makes the following reflections:

> Mohammed has suffered recurrent existential crises in his life, resulting in an erosion of his sense of self-mastery and social worth that he has tried to make good by calling upon beliefs in shape- shifting. As an elephant he is in his element, empowered by a sense of amplitude and control. But as with alcohol and drug use in our society, Mohammed's clandestine gains are at the cost of social integration. His vicarious mastery of the world entails, ironically, a separation from it, a marginality whose ambivalent images are those of solitude, sorcery, and the bush.
>
> The situation brings to mind the Kuranko women who confess to being witches during serious illness, calling upon the stereotypes of witchcraft to comprehend and cope with a crisis that erodes self-control and subverts identity. As in the case of shape-shifters, the confession is socially useful, affirming the veracity of witchcraft beliefs, but self-defeating, for unless she dies of natural causes the self-confessed witch may be ritually killed.
>
> (Jackson 2012: 105)

Dealing with evil spirits among machi is more ambiguous than shape-shifting among the Kuranko. This is to say that, although it is a source of moral ambiguity and, thus, isolation and marginality, treating evil spirits is also a source of wealth and power. In turn, wealth and power can be used as a constructive force in the sense that they can integrate an individual into the social group. For instance, a machi can use their money to organize a community ritual event (and I observed some of them doing so). Therefore, these clandestine gains are not necessarily only self-defeating as shape- shifting beliefs were for Mohammed. Machi who deal effectively with evil spirits and witchcraft enhance their reputation among patients and receive generous monetary compensation. As witchcraft and evil spirits are invisible to biomedical methods of disease detection, the capacity of making evil spirits visible gives machi a field of action free of competition from other health practitioners. In fact, many of my informants told me that because machi are the only type of people who can see evil spirits, machi should continue to exist.

Witchcraft is the main reason why non-Mapuche people seek the help of a machi. Machi exploit their own exoticism and otherness as a source of power when dealing with occult forces. At the same time, machi's exoticism is the result of a colonial encounter, which both marginalized and created new sources of clandestine power. In his ethnography on the Indigenous people of Putumayo River in south-eastern Colombia, Taussig (1986) argues that Europeans introduced *magia* (magic) to the region in the seventeenth century. European missionaries strongly believed in witchcraft, and they considered Indigenous people prone to it given their pact with the devil (ibid.: 142–43). To prevent white people from going to Indigenous healers, missionaries violently prohibited the performance of Indigenous healing rituals. But Taussig argued that this violent repression confirmed white people's beliefs in the power of Indigenous healers.

> Yet was not the diabolic memory here at issue that of the Spanish and not of the Indians? The momentous irony was that in struggling to erase these "memories," the Church was in fact creating and strengthening them as a new social force, thereby ensuring the transmission of myth into reality and memory into the future.
>
> (Taussig 1986: 143)

In discussing the ritual event of searching for the *entierro*, I have tried to highlight the relevance of techniques of seeing in ritual performative efficacy. By generating communal seeing, machi generate an objectifying and exteriorizing experience of evil spirits that prepares individuals for effective ritual action. Seeing the evil spirits confirms the cause of the affliction and weakens the evil agent so it can be effectively expelled. While the ritual described in this section constitutes a witchcraft practice, the case described below does not involve the evil acts of a witch. Moreover, in what follows, the treatment of evil spirits is assumed as an opportunity to confront the sick person with her own responsibility regarding her health. Gradually, conversations shifted from evil agents of illness to family negotiations of mutual care and responsibility. However, techniques of seeing evil spirits remained fundamental to ritual performative efficacy.

The *Ulutun* Ritual

In this case, the relationship between the machi and the patient did not originate from the recommendations of other patients. Rather, the machi and the patient's daughter, Olga, were close friends and shared a long-lasting relationship of mutual commitment. In this way, Olga asked the machi to visit her mother, who was sick, as a healer/friend.

Olga and the machi belonged to the same Indigenous community and lived close to each other (about ten minutes by foot). Neither of them was born in the community they now considered their own. Olga had arrived there after getting married and the machi, along with her husband, had decided to buy land there and moved in about eight years before I met them. For Olga, the arrival of the machi and her husband changed things in the community for the better. "Since she arrived, we [the community] do things together. Now, we celebrate the *nguillatun*. Only after she came did we start celebrating the *ngillatun*. When I came to live here, people did not celebrate the *nguillatun* and they did not care about their culture. Also, people respect traditional ceremonies now and men do not get drunk. That is also thanks to the machi, she is very strict," Olga told me. For Olga, the machi was a friend but not an ordinary one, since she thought her friend was keeping the community together and bringing back the respect and interest in traditional ceremonies. Therefore, the machi was a figure of authority, community and belonging.

The house of the machi in Olga's community was a frequent meeting place. Olga and other members of her community gathered there to plan social events, such as birthday parties and trips to the beach, as well as political negotiations with the municipality and other forms of local government. Also, at the machi's house, people gathered to organize the *ngillatun* ritual and other community ceremonies. Thus, the machi's house was a place to discuss social, political and religious issues. Moreover, Olga and other close friends assisted the machi with performing healing rituals and preparing herbal infusions for patients. The machi paid her friends who helped her as *keyu* (assistants) in cash. In this way, a successful healer in a community is also an opportunity for occasional paid work.

Olga turned to the machi in cases of illness and misfortune, like most other people in her community did. "We know she will help us. She is generous and only ask for small donations in return. Sometimes, she does not even ask for that. We are very lucky we have a machi in our community. We know we must take care of her in return," Olga told me. Members of the community constantly visited or called the machi by phone to ask for health advice. In case of emergency, calls and visits could occur in the middle of the night.

The machi was always willing to attend to patients and even more so if they were friends and members of her community.

In this way, Olga and the machi shared a long relationship of mutual commitment as friends, neighbors and members of the same Indigenous community. In addition, Olga turned to the machi in cases of illness, while the machi turned to Olga if she needed assistance with her duties as a healer. This is a kind of relationship between a machi and a friend/patient that leads people to refer to a machi as "my machi." In this way, a person speaks of "my machi" when they go to the machi in cases of illness, collaborates with the machi as an assistant, participates in the same *ngillatun* ceremony, or considers the machi a friend. In turn, machi encourage people to refer to them in such a way. For example, when I visited a machi after being away for a while, she told me: "I thought you had forgotten your machi." Implicitly, this idiom implies that people should only seek the help of one machi and remain loyal to them. In practice, people do tend to go to the same machi over long periods of time. However, if symptoms or problems persist, they usually go to more than one machi.

Olga's mother, Rosa, was an elderly woman in her late sixties, who lived in the mountains of the Araucanía region (about seventy miles east of Olga's house). Rosa lived with her husband, one of her daughters and her grandson (an eight-year-old boy). Olga explained to me why she was asking her machi to visit her mother. A few months earlier, Rosa started acting in an odd way. She was aggressive and erratic, she did not sleep at night, and she was experiencing "visions" and "disorientation." At one point she lost consciousness and was taken by her family to the nearest hospital. Rosa was hospitalized and diagnosed with a diabetic coma. During her hospitalization she was stabilized, and insulin was initiated. When she returned home from the hospital, she was still feeling tired and nervous. According to Olga, Rosa was reacting irritably toward her family and did not cooperate with the strict diet prescribed for her. She passively accepted the insulin injections that she needed during the day but delegated all responsibility to Olga's younger sister. Thus, Rosa showed no interest in learning the schedules or doses of insulin injections, or much less, in learning to inject herself.

I drove Olga and the machi to Rosa's place on a cold morning in June. During that first visit we stayed for an entire day. We arrived at lunchtime and left the following day right after lunch. The machi was there as a healer and as a friend. Conversations referred to a variety of topics such as talking about their mutual friends, asking about family members who were not there, asking me questions and getting to know why I was there, the coming celebration of the Mapuche New Year, among other things. We ate together and spent most of the time chatting at the dining table. However, we also had a walk around the farm. Olga was proud of showing me the "most beautiful volcano of the world," the Llaima volcano, which we could impressively see from her parents' land.

Throughout the day, members of the family expressed their concerns. Olga and her sister were worried about their mother because they thought Rosa was acting in a moody and childish manner. For example, Rosa insisted on leaving the house although the weather was cold, and doctors had advised her not to do so (Rosa was recovering from pneumonia as well as a diabetic decompensation). Moreover, she was boycotting the diet, either by not eating at all (which can be dangerous after an insulin dose due to the risk of hypoglycemia) or eating secretly what she was not supposed to. Olga also said that she felt her mother was weak, aged, and incapable of reassuming her home duties. Rosa's husband, José, had to assume responsibility for household activities, while the younger daughter worked during the day. The daughters also resented the fact that Rosa knew she had diabetes prior to her hospitalization. Nevertheless, Rosa did not comply with the treatment. She simply did not take the oral drugs she was prescribed (these drugs are provided free of charge at local primary care centers). Now it was too late, the drugs were useless, and Rosa depended on her insulin doses.

Rosa was worried about the effects diabetes may have on her body. When she realized I was a doctor she asked me many questions about diabetes: Can it be cured? Will I end up blind? Will I end up needing dialysis? Rosa told me that her sister had also had the disease and had died during dialysis. She told me, in a sad and anxious tone, that her sister had suffered greatly. The stay at the hospital had been traumatic for Rosa and she complained about negligent treatment on the part of the nursing staff. The hospitalization had left her feeling exhausted and defeated.

Besides medical and social concerns, Rosa also expressed spiritual worries. She told us that not long before the diabetes coma occurred, she went to a *zatun* ritual, which is a healing ritual in which a machi diagnoses and treats illnesses through trance, music, medicinal herbs, and massage (described in detail in Chapter 4). A neighbor was sick, and Rosa was asked by the sick man's family to participate in the ritual. Usually when conducting a *zatun* ritual people ask for the help of family, neighbors, and friends. Rosa went on to say that, during trance, the machi who officiated the ceremony shouted angrily at the sick man, accusing him of being an alcoholic and beating his wife. Rosa left the ceremony feeling emotionally impacted by these revelations concerning her neighbors' private family life. After listening to Rosa's story, the machi proposed the hypothesis, which Rosa and her family had already been contemplating, that the evil that affected Rosa's neighbor had been transferred from the neighbor to Rosa's body. Because Rosa was sick, she was vulnerable to evil spirits. In Mapudungun this is called a *konün* (a verb that means "to enter" but is used here as a noun), which means that an evil spirit is transferred from one body to another, usually more vulnerable, one. The machi who officiated the ceremony Rosa attended acted negligently or simply did not have enough power to neutralize the evil spirit he was dealing with. Therefore, Rosa was a victim of human irresponsibility in dealing with evil spirits they are not prepared to face. At the same time, Rosa was responsible for neglecting the treatment of the disease that made her vulnerable to evil spirits (i.e., diabetes).

At night, the machi performed a cleansing (S: *limpieza*) of the house. Having asserted that the probable origin of disease was an evil spirit, the machi then needed to keep evil forces at bay. Holding a fire pit in which counterhex herbs were burning, the machi went through each room of the house, as well as through the immediate surroundings of the house (which was on a plot of approximately five hectares), commanding, in Mapudungun, that the evil spirits leave. When the machi went out of the house with Rosa's husband and daughters, I stayed inside the house with Rosa, who was not allowed to go out. Rosa looked tense and worried. She kept asking me if they had really gone through all the rooms in the house. Suddenly, everybody came back looking very agitated. "We have seen it!" they said. They had seen a shadow with a human form running away from them. "You should have come," the machi said to me. They had really seen it, they explained, as you can see the shadow of an animal or a person moving in the middle of the night.

In this way, the machi constructed the stage that made the ritual healing described below necessary. In other words, she constructed the diagnosis on her first visit and later came back to treat the patient on her second visit. The machi patiently took a whole day to listen to each member of the family express their concerns. After listening, she proposed an explanation of the problems Rosa continued to face: an evil spirit entered Rosa's body when she attended a healing ceremony officiated by an irresponsible machi. The diabetes made Rosa vulnerable to evil spirits, but it was the spirit that almost killed her. Therefore, the machi needed to "clean" the house of evil influences through performing a *sahumerio* (burning incense) and praying. While conducting these actions they saw the evil spirit; that is, the diagnosis was confirmed just as visual imagery confirmed an evil spirit was causing the affliction in the ritual of searching for the *entierro*. To effectively expel the evil spirit, the machi needed to carry out a more complex ritual. Again, after seeing the evil spirit and, thus, confirming its negative impact on a person's health, ritual action against it can be properly initiated. It was decided that they were going to wait for better weather to perform the healing ritual needed since the machi explained that they could not perform this ritual inside the house and Rosa was still too weak to leave the house (as doctors had advised).

As promised, the machi returned to perform the healing ritual prescribed two months after the initial visit. We arrived in the evening when it was already dark. This time the machi arrived with an assistant (who was also Olga's friend and neighbor), Olga, and I. Rosa's family had asked two men who were her husband's nephews and lived nearby to assist them with the ceremony. In addition, they had also asked for the help of a close friend and her daughter. Unlike the first visit, in which the machi conversed on different topics and walked across the field to enjoy the view of the Llaima volcano, on this second occasion the machi immediately came to carry out the healing ritual. She went straight into action.

The family had prepared a ground-floor storage room in which the healing would occur. It was a wooden room about three meters square, separated from the house. In the center of the room a mattress was placed, with the head facing a door that was facing east. A large brazier was put near the mattress, so Rosa would not get cold and the machi could burn counterhexes. Two *foye* tree (canelo or winter's bark) branches were placed in two large flowerpots, one at the head and the other at the foot of the mattress. Rosa's husband, together with the other two men, had previously gathered and cut the branches. Olga had gathered *lawen* (medicinal plants), such as *maqui* (Chilean wineberry) and *foye*. These plants are believed to be protectors against evil spirits. The medicinal leaves were placed in wicker baskets at the foot of the mattress.

When we arrived, Rosa was already on the mattress, covered with several blankets, and remained there throughout most of the healing ceremony. The two men, Rosa's nephews, were standing on both sides of the patient's head holding a *wiño* (wooden canes used in the *palin* game and in traditional ceremonies), as guardians holding their arms. The head of the patient was facing an open door that was facing east. Just outside the door, two other large branches of *foye* (canelo) had been planted in the earth. In that place healing actions began. The participants knelt before the *foye* branches. The first action was a *llellipun* (prayer) accompanied by the *kultrun* (ritual drum) and *kaskawilla* (a ribbon or leather band tied to the hand, to which bronze jingle bells are attached). During the prayer, the machi and family members asked *Ngenechen* (God) to allow Rosa to recover her health, free her from the action of evil spirits and return her to her loved ones who were waiting for her.

After the initial prayer, the machi entered the room where the patient was lying and spat *aguardiente* (a grape distillate with high alcohol content) everywhere to keep away evil spirits. Then, she started playing her *kultrun* and dancing while she chanted, to continue to ask for the health of the patient, while commanding evil spirits to leave. She danced around the patient's body, and we all encouraged her, playing the *kaskawilla* and animating her with the *afafan* (ritual shout of encouragement). The two men who were holding the *wiño* beat them against each other. The machi handed her *kultrun* to her assistant, who continued to play while the machi continued chanting as she started to massage the body of the patient. The massage (S: *friega*) was done by rubbing medicinal herbs against all parts of the patient's body. She did it in an energetic way, but at the same time she was careful to massage each part of the body and cover with the blankets the parts that she had already massaged. The machi also inhaled cigar smoke and exhaled it over the body of the patient on repeated occasions.

While inhaling and exhaling cigar smoke, the machi proceeded to go out of the room where the patient was, to "clean" the surroundings with the smoke of the cigars. She asked where it was exactly that they had seen the shadow with a human form the last time she had been there. Rosa's husband took her there, where she addressed the evil spirit, commanding it to leave the house so that Rosa could recover. The machi was always followed by the two men holding the *wiño,* who were required to act as protectors. When she came back to the patient, she massaged her again while the rest of the participants continued to play music. When she finished, the machi asked to be brought a branch of *Espino*, which is a branch with thorns. With those branches she slammed the walls of the room in which we were and then went outside of the room to keep hitting the walls from the outside. From inside the wooden room, the blows could be heard and, during one of them, the light went out, an event that caused expressions of fear. An ampule hung from the ceiling and illuminated the inside of the storage room. When extinguished, in one of the many hits to the wall that the machi gave, we were completely in the dark, except for the faint light radiating from the embers of the brazier. The men hurried to make the light come back on, while the machi did not stop, not even for a minute, to slam the walls of the room. When the bulb again illuminated over our heads, the machi stopped and asked the whole group, "Who is the person who saw it?" Her assistant immediately responded that she had heard the voice of a child shouting, "Help me!" She felt the child's voice so close to one of her ears that the ear was now burning. Olga said she had seen a child running and shouting, "Help me!" As I described for the ritual of searching for the *entierro*, these experiences are immediately understood as the presence of an evil spirit. Therefore, they are confirmation that an evil force is causing the decline in Rosa's health. In addition, these visual and auditory images are an indication that ritual action is weakening the evil spirit by exteriorizing it.

Rosa was lifted from the mattress and dressed in dry clothes. When she was dressed, the machi threw some "secret herbs" into the brazier, which caused a large amount of smoke that made it difficult to breathe, as it irritated the throat. It also made it difficult to see because the smoke blurred our vision. Everybody was coughing and crying, which caused the laughter of some, and somewhat playful questions to the machi, such as, "What the hell does this *sahumerio* [burning incense] have?" The intoxicating smoke of the *sahumerio* harnessed the participants' body against the action of evil spirits, just as the aroma of herbs and incense, the chanting voice of the machi, and the smell and taste of the *aguardiente* did when people were preparing to search for the *entierro*.

As a closing moment to the ceremony, we all greeted and welcomed Rosa back, wishing her strength and health. The machi instructed that we should welcome Rosa back from sickness and encourage her to be strong and recover. The machi was the first one who performed a welcome back to Rosa. After observing what the machi did, we all knew how to welcome Rosa back from sickness. The machi hugged and kissed Rosa while saying "*newentulei, lamgen*" (be strong, sister). The machi then grabbed José and pushed him toward his wife. José hugged and kissed Rosa and said, "Be strong, I need you back." The couple remained in each other's arms for a while. When Rosa separated from her husband, Olga was right next to her waiting for her turn to greet and welcome her back. When mother and daughter hugged and kissed each other there were tears on their faces. The younger daughter did as her father and sister had done, while the rest of us waited in line for our turn to hug Rosa and give words of encouragement and hope. It was a moving welcoming of a family to a member who had almost died, and a verbalization of the hope that she would be healthy again, that she was going to be who she had always been: their wife, mother, grandmother, aunt, and friend.

The ceremony required about two hours of demanding physical work. After it was finished, we came back inside the house and sat around the dining table, while Rosa's daughters started serving food. The conversation that followed continued until three o'clock in the morning. People restated what they had seen and heard. Olga and Rosa had seen a child running, the machi's assistant heard a child shouting "help me" into her ear, more people had seen the figure of a child. Rosa's friend said she had not seen anything, in a tone of disbelief. She was ignored by the rest of the participants, who continued their conversation about what they had seen. When we had finished eating, the implements used in the ceremony, such as cigars, medicinal leaves, blankets, and *Espino* branches, were taken to the nearest river and thrown into it. Through this action, the evil spirit is finally disposed of, leaving the people and their living space "clean."

Rosa was a victim of chaotic forces disturbing her body and thoughts. Treatment, then, needed to re-establish a sense of self-control and agency. The person needs to restore their body limits to recover their own characteristic ways of relating and being, as well as their connections and obligations within a system of relations. Regaining a sense of self-control is actively achieved during ritual action. The body is awakened through different forms of sensory engagement such as music, chants, burning incense, and massage. In addition, external demonic influences are "seen" or made into a lived experience through ritual techniques. Thus, they become something that can be grasped by the senses. In other words, through the involvement of imagination the evil spirit becomes an indexical sign in the form of a child's scream in the ear, an ear burning or visualizing a child running. The evil spirit is seen and felt through the senses and the circulation of shared emotional states. In this way, ritual action creates the experience of the liberation of demonic forces through the involvement of the senses, the imagination and the emotions. To be able to have that experience is essential for ritual performative efficacy, so the machi insists that everybody needs "to see." Appealing to sight gives undeniable connotation of reality to the experience and avoids any dichotomy between real or imagined, perception or sensation. If people engage in this kind of disquisition, the ritual loses efficacy. Therefore, Rosa's friend's experience of not seeing anything was ignored. Thus, the machi created for Rosa the conditions necessary to experience the recovery of agency and self-control, together with the return from sickness and the hospital to her family and network of connections. Therefore, agency and personal ways of being are restored, while belonging to a family and social relations is transformed into a lived experience. Hugs, kisses, loving words, and emotive tears welcomed Rosa back to her family and social ties.

The conversation people had also addressed Rosa's responsibility toward herself. Her family said she had to take care of her body, she had to follow her diet. She also needed to recognize how difficult her disease had been for everybody. Her husband, an old man, had assumed household duties, while still taking care of the animals and the farm. Her daughter cooked separately for her, even though it meant a double job. The daughter also learned all her insulin schedules, doses and glycemic controls. Rosa protested that her diet was tasteless. She asked for time to get used to it. She also asked her family to understand that she did not want to be locked up in the house all the time. People shared ideas about better food for diabetic patients and where to obtain it. The family members also agreed that Rosa would go to a birthday party that was coming soon; they were finally willing to let Rosa reinitiate her social life outside her home.

To be back in her social position and role, Rosa must take responsibility. She must actively act again not only as a person in control of herself, but also as a person with obligations that are moral and affective ties. José told her: "I want you to want to live again." This phrase caused more tears in Rosa's eyes. It was the verbalization of Rosa's fear that diabetes would make her life miserable, as she thought had happened to her sister. Her willingness to live and survive the disease episode was constructed through the recovery of both her individuality and agency, and the sense of belonging to a network of relationships to which she was morally and affectively tied.

We only slept for three hours, because the ritual actions needed to be repeated before sunrise. We woke up at six o'clock in the morning to carry out the ceremony again. Although we were tired, the actions were carefully repeated in a second event that lasted an hour. We then left early after breakfast. I came back to visit Rosa the following month. She was feeling better and looked younger. She had regained confidence in her strength and was again in charge of home duties. She was baking the bread for her family almost every day, as she had always done before she became sick, which gave her a sense of pride and self-worth.

In discussing different techniques to see evil spirits, I have shown how aspects of ritual healing transformations occur at a pre-symbolic level. Furthermore, pre-symbolic sensory and affective transformations are essential for ritual performative efficacy for at least the following reasons. First, they promote imaginative and creative engagement with an existential situation through the induction of synchronicity or communal seeing. Second, as they are shared by a group of participants, they produce the sense of acting together that can mobilize affective dispositions and attenuate interpersonal conflict. Lastly, the performative seeing, search for, and disposal of evil spirits can promote fruitful negotiations of mutual moral and affective responsibilities.

Notes

1. On one occasion, I witnessed the celebration of a *ngillatun* ritual in which some authorities of CONADI were invited. CONADI bought the ancestral ceremonial site in which the ceremony took place. The ceremonial site used to be in private hands (it belonged to one of the members of the Indigenous community) and it was being used to cultivate the land. CONADI bought the land so it could become the collective property of the Indigenous community again. In this way, it was possible to resume the celebration of the *ngillatun* in that place, which had been interrupted for years after the division and privatization of Indigenous land. This example shows the privileged status of some Mapuche cultural practices, such as the *ngillatun* ritual, in the eyes of the Chilean state. It also shows how Mapuche leaders engage in acts of reciprocity with state authorities through the participation in some events of Mapuche ritual life.
2. The *ulutun* ritual is usually performed at a machi's house and it is commonly described by my informants as a shorter version of a *zatun* ritual (described in Chapter 4). Unlike the *zatun* ritual, the *ulutun* ritual does not involve ritual trance. In addition, the *ulutun* ritual is usually carried out with the machi and the patient as the sole participants. The healing actions (drumming, massaging, praying, and divining through *pewtun* techniques) need to be performed twice: once at dusk and a second time at dawn. The patient usually sleeps at the machi's home. The ritual described here may be described as an *ulutun* ritual, but it seems highly idiosyncratic. It preserves the general structure but includes innovations and improvisations. Bacigalupo (2001: 87) referred to the *ulutun* ritual as a possible recent innovation in which the machi does not enter into trance but chants and massages (S: *friega*) the patient with medicinal herbs. It is also significantly cheaper than a *zatun* ritual (ibid.: 88).
3. The machi speech in *pewtun* sessions described in Chapter 2 builds uncertainty as described here.
4. This technique resembles how Catholic Charismatic healers inculcate visual imagery through the "shoe test" as described in Chapter 1 (Csordas 1994a: 76).
5. Csordas (1994a: 109) understands ritual efficacy as transforming the self, while therapeutic efficacy consists of alleviating suffering. In the Catholic Charismatic context, the latter is strictly complementary to the former. In the case described here, I propose that they are not necessarily complementary.
6. The ambiguous position of the victim of evil has been highlighted in the anthropological literature. Stroeken (2008) described how, when bewitched, "people become hunted by the idea of an unpaid debt" (ibid.: 475), due to which an ancestor or a member of the family has turned against them after feeling offended. Whyte (1997) described that when people go to see a diviner to discover who has caused their misfortune, the divination "involves moral reflections not only about the agent [the witch], but about the victim and the people responsible for the victim … a divination bears certain resemblance to a court trial" (ibid.: 32). Favret-Saada (1980) described a case in which the victim of witchcraft was originally the suspected witch.

Chapter 4
Machi Who Are Not Real Machi
Doubts and Failure

In Chapter 2, two requisites were proposed as necessary in order to be considered a real machi: to see illnesses and misfortunes through different therapeutic techniques and to preside over collective ceremonies in a convincing manner. At a doctrinal level, a real machi is one who has a machi lineage spirit and remains in permanent communication with it through dreams, visions, intuition, and ritual trance. Here, I explore two cases in which machi are not perceived as real, or at least doubts regarding their authenticity or efficacy are voiced by some people. The first case concerns a middle-aged machi, Ana, whose spirit had abandoned her, leaving her powerless and sick. To make the spirit return to the machi's body, a healing ritual was performed. The machi's performance during the ritual event left some members of the audience unconvinced regarding the efficacy of the ritual and, more significantly, the authenticity of the machi herself. The second case refers to a *machil* (machi initiate), Marta, who is unable to divine or preside over ceremonies because she thinks she is not yet prepared and fears making a mistake. Thus, she cannot become a machi and her initiation process remains incomplete. In the first case, skepticism regarding the machi's powers originates in a perceived imperfect performance by some of the participants of a ritual event. In contrast, the second case illustrates an inability to perform in the first place. Marta does not doubt she has a machi spirit and, thus, she is a real lineage machi, but she does doubt that she could be efficacious as a healer because she cannot interpret her spirit's messages. Her doubts prevent her from performing as a healer, even after an initiation ritual event was perceived as efficacious by most of the participants; that is, Marta's spirit was made present through ritual trance, confirming that Marta was indeed chosen by her spirit and could become a machi.

A Failed Performance: A Machi Who Was Not Really in Trance

Although ineffective ritual treatment has been explored in medical anthropology (e.g., Hüsken 2007; Lewis 2000; Schieffelin 1996), it has probably drawn less attention as a topic of research than therapeutic processes and events perceived as efficacious. One of the reasons this may be the case is that ritual is considered sacred and, thus, infallible at a doctrinal level: people can fail, but not the spirits or the gods. This is the case among the Mapuche, for whom, when things go wrong, the moral and spiritual integrity of the healer or the patient is at stake but not the ritual itself.[1] But regardless of where failure lies, within the ritual itself or the performers or the relationship with the broader context, failure is, indeed, a possible outcome for any ritual event.

Another reason why failure of treatment has not been systematically explored may be that failure is a morally loaded word that implies a moral accusation. Therefore, ethnographers may be reluctant to use the term. Schieffelin (2007) proposed to use the term "imperfection" instead of failure, observing that ritual performances are rarely interrupted or abandoned altogether despite mishaps and mistakes.[2] In this way, imperfect rituals refer to "rites which do their job acceptably but don't do it well: e.g. not without conflict, or not without correction or not to everyone's satisfaction, or not in proper style – but don't actually fail" (ibid.: 16–17). Contrarily, failure should be reserved for where "ritual breaks down, loses its authority or becomes discredited" (ibid.: 16). In the case discussed here, the ritual performance was not interrupted, the healer was not confronted, and only some people, but not all, were severely dissatisfied with the performance. In that sense, one could say that the performance was imperfect rather than a total failure. However, as an ethnographer, one should be careful not to underestimate the social consequences of perceived failure, even if failure is partial and inconclusive.[3] While most ritual mistakes and mishaps are ignored or corrected during or after ritual action and do not compromise the authenticity of the performers and the perceived efficacy of the ritual, in this case the healer's mistakes did seem to damage her reputation. To fully grasp the very real consequences of perceived failure in the context of ritual healing is in line with the idea that ritual has the potential to change people's circumstances for better or worse.

In the analysis of the case presented here, I understand ritual failure as a performance failure (Grimes 1990; Schieffelin 1996, 2007). In turn, performance failure can be defined as procedural errors and mishaps or as unusual and unexpected events that change a particular ritual performance (Schieffelin 2007: 4–7). One of the most important things at stake in a Mapuche ritual healing performance is the authenticity of the machi. Particularly significant to the identification of this is the moment of trance, since this is the moment in which the spirits are made present. While in trance, a machi is possessed by their spirit, who gives information regarding prevention, identification, and treatment of illnesses and problems. On the occasion discussed here, doubts were raised regarding the authenticity of the trance and, thus, the presence of the machi spirit and the effectiveness of the ritual. The machi committed several procedural mistakes, but it was the deployment of an improper emotion while in trance (the machi cried) that affected how her performance was perceived.

Machi Ana's Illness

Machi Ana was a married woman in her late fifties who lived in a rural Mapuche community with her husband and two daughters. She worked as a Mapuche healer in a local state-sponsored Mapuche medical center and she also treated patients privately at her home. Every time I visited her at her home, in the morning, there were two or three patients waiting for her to perform a uroscopy. The people who worked with her at the Mapuche medical center considered her far less popular than other machi. In addition, Machi Ana was not being invited to preside over *ngillatun* rituals. Moreover, the machi's own community had stopped celebrating the *ngillatun* ritual because most of its members had converted to Pentecostalism.

Machi Ana had various chronic diseases, such as diabetes, hypertension, and osteoarthritis, for which she received medications at the local rural medical post.[4] She was usually in pain and used to walk with some difficulty due to this. When discussing her health problems with colleagues at the Mapuche medical center where she worked, Machi Ana told her colleagues that "my spirit has left me, I am weak, I have lost power." She added that it was not only that she was feeling tired and weak, but also that she had lost her ability to treat sick people effectively. This is a very serious admission for a machi to make and one that could compromise her credibility as a healer. In the same conversation, Machi Ana asked her colleagues for support. She explained she needed to perform a *zatun* ritual to recover her health and her abilities as a machi. For such a ritual to be effective, the machi needed the participation of as many people as possible. Thus, the machi was asking her colleagues to participate in the ritual and to ask members of their families to participate as well.

Machi Ana's condition was severe enough to need the help of another "compatible" machi. Machi Rosalía was chosen as a healer by Machi Ana and her family. Machi Rosalía had been treating Machi Ana with herbal remedies after performing several sessions of uroscopy. Eventually she also agreed to perform a *zatun* ritual.

Machi Ana explained that the reason her spirit had left her, leaving her weak and sick, was *wezanewen,* or negative energies. She thought that evil spiritual forces had taken control over her body, moving her away from her machi spirit. Those evil forces originated in deliberate acts to provoke harm. Ana thought other machi considered her a rival or a competitor and were trying to get rid of the competition by using witchcraft against her. She blamed a machi with whom she officiated a ceremony in a community close to her own a year before I met her. According to Ana, this other machi prevented her from going into trance, expelling her spirit when it was about to come. As Ana could not go into trance, the other machi took control of the ceremony. In fact, after that incident, Ana had not returned to preside over any ceremony, since no community had requested it. In addition, she had not experienced trance again.

Interestingly, Machi Rosalía had a somehow different version regarding the cause of Ana's affliction. As was usual among the machi I worked with, Machi Rosalía was inclined to emphasize Ana's responsibility both in causing her illness and in recovering from it. Rosalía thought Machi Ana was not behaving in a way expected of a machi. Thus, Ana's spirit was angry and was trying to make her change. When I asked Rosalía what it was that Ana was doing wrong, she detailed the following: Ana was not playing her ritual drum every morning; the ritual drum was too old, and its sound was not the proper one; she had not renovated the branches and flags of her *rewe* (altar). Because the machi spirit had left, Ana was weak and vulnerable to natural diseases, like the ones described above, namely hypertension, diabetes, and osteoarthritis. In addition, Ana was vulnerable to the acts of evil spirits. According to Machi Rosalía, Machi Ana not only needed to chase away evil spirits, but she also needed to change her behavior to convince her spirit to return and continue to give her the strength to treat illness. Only a change in her own behavior could protect Ana against evil spirits and natural diseases, as well as give her back her machi powers. To Rosalía, the *zatun* ritual was necessary because it could give the sick machi instructions from her spirit as to what was expected from her. "We will talk with the spirits and then she will know what to do," machi Rosalía told me. In this way, each machi emphasized the causes of Ana's affliction differently. While Machi Ana posited the responsibility on the evil actions of envious people, Machi Rosalía highlighted Ana's own responsibility in her spirit rejecting her and the need for a change in her conduct.

There are many reasons that can explain why a machi is attacked by an evil force. These reasons are usually related to moral transgressions, deliberate or unconscious, self-produced or produced by a third person (usually a member of the family, even from a past generation). Then, Machi Ana could have transgressed her own responsibilities as a healing person in many ways: being a witch (using her powers to harm people); not using the proper utensils during a healing ritual or the proper *lawen* (medicine) a person needed; treating patients she was not compatible with; performing a ritual when there were not enough people there or no proper preparation had been made; failing to recognize that she would not cure a specific person; and other mistakes. If she fails to carry out her obligations as a healing person, her spirit can turn its back on her, making her vulnerable to attacks from evil spirits. Or her machi spirit may cause symptoms and misfortunes to provoke a change in her conduct. Then, every time a machi engages in medical and ritual action, they are risking severe consequences if they make a mistake. "Maybe a patient came to her and she did not tell him that she was not going to be able to cure him. She decided to take the risk and the disease transferred to her," a man told me, referring to Machi Ana's health problems.

Other people who participated in the ritual thought that Ana's family was responsible for her ill health. Both her husband and her daughters were not sufficiently involved in her machi practice. In addition to the disinterest of her family, Ana also faced the rejection of the people in her community. Most families in Ana's community had converted to Pentecostalism, thus they considered Mapuche medical practices as diabolic. Therefore, Machi Ana did not have support either from her family or from her community. However, some people also thought that part of the responsibility fell on Ana herself. I was told there were rumors about Ana's past. Some believed she used to use black magic in exchange for money. Machi Ana and her family had experienced the sudden and tragic loss of family members on two occasions. The origin of such misfortune could be Ana's own morally reproachable conduct as a machi. I observed that the occurrence of tragic events in a family usually generated suspicions about the moral integrity of that family. Moreover, some people told me that most people living near Ana feared she was a witch. Thus, she was not invited to preside over community ceremonies.

The Zatun *Ritual*

The *zatun* ritual is the most complex healing ritual carried out by machi from the sixteenth century until today.[5] The ritual usually takes place at the sick person's home and involves the participation of family, friends, and neighbors. It requires the use of considerable social and economic resources. Nowadays, the cost varies greatly. Some machi may charge up to 500,000 Chilean pesos (US$840) for performing a *zatun* ritual. However, a family would need to spend far more money than just the machi's fees. This is because they need to feed all the participants and perform the proper preparations. Thus, a family can easily part with about a million Chilean pesos (US$1,600) for a ceremony. Some machi, though, charge much less. In the event described here, Machi Rosalía only charged 50,000 Chilean pesos (US$84).

The ritual usually starts at nightfall, and it is repeated at dawn. In between the two parts, the participants go to sleep in the sick person's home. A *zatun* ritual consists of prayers, chants, massage, and trance. The first ceremony is usually followed by dinner and the second one by breakfast. Hosts usually offer meat, potatoes, bread, red wine, and *mate* tea in abundance to their guests. The people necessary for the healing ritual to take place are, at least, the following: the machi and a *zugumachife* (ritual interpreter), *llancan*, (ritual dancers, usually one female and one male) and musicians; the patient and their family and close friends (M: *ngen kutran*). The patient's family is responsible for feeding the participants and providing the machi with most of the ritual paraphernalia. The machi and their assistants are responsible for leading the ritual performance. Usually, families invite relatives, friends and neighbors to participate. In the event discussed here around forty people participated.

Machi Ana's house was situated on top of a chain of hills overlooking the coastline, where you could feel the sea breeze. As usual in Mapuche communities, the nearest neighbor's house was barely visible. Despite the feeling of isolation that the place produced, the roads leading there were well cared for and, to a large extent, paved. Therefore, it was relatively easy to access the property, even during the winter, which was the time of year in which this ritual occurred. I drove there from the nearest town, and the drive lasted only about thirty minutes. As was the case with many people's plot of land, Ana's property had a relatively new and well-kept subsidy house and next to it an old wooden house. People do not demolish old dwellings when they build a new one. Rather, they keep using old houses as storerooms, kitchens, or places to accommodate guests. What indicated the presence of a machi in that house was the *rewe* (altar) in the middle of the courtyard.

The day of the ceremony, I arrived at Machi Ana's home at 6:15 a.m. I went there with a group of friends who worked together with the machi at a local Mapuche medical center. When we arrived at the machi's house, there were several people, approximately twenty, performing various tasks. More people continued to arrive throughout the morning, including Machi Rosalía and her assistants. Several men were driving across the countryside looking for large branches of native trees to dress the *rewe* (altar). Other men were using *coligüe* sticks to make new blue and white flags to put in the *rewe*. Inside the house, several women were making bread and cooking meat to offer breakfast to the participants. We were served breakfast by female friends and relatives of the machi. We ate bread, fried bread (S: *sopaipillas*), chicken, and eggs. *Vino harinao* or *chupilca* (red wine mixed with toasted flour and sugar) was also offered. Machi Ana was seated at her kitchen table with her guests, chatting about the state of her health. She was feeling weak and experiencing nausea, therefore, she was not able to eat.

Machi Rosalía arrived at 8:30 a.m. in a van that Ana's family had rented for the occasion. A male friend of the family was driving the van. The two machi, Ana and Rosalía, lived approximately fifteen miles away from each other. Rosalía came with five other people including her husband, father-in-law, brother-in-law and his wife, and a young man who was a friend and neighbor. Machi Rosalía and her assistants were served breakfast. Her presence increased the pressure to finish the preparations so that the ceremony could begin.

After breakfast, Rosalía started to prepare the place for the ceremony. She began inside the house, where she placed a mattress just inside of the entrance door, in a room that was used as a living and dining room and kitchen. The door of the house remained wide open throughout the ceremony. Next to the mattress, at its head, Rosalía placed a small bench onto which a white tablecloth was put. On the bench, Rosalía placed a jug of clay with spring water, another with *mote* or boiled grains of wheat, and a third one with *muday* (a beverage made by fermenting grains of wheat). A jug of clay containing *aguardiente* (grape distillate) and another one with red wine in it were also placed on the bench, beside shotgun cartridges and cigarettes. Next to the small bench, a small chair was placed, where Machi Rosalía was later going to be seated during the initial part of the ritual.

A wicker basket filled with leaves of medicinal plants was placed at the foot of the mattress. The medicinal leaves had been previously gathered by Ana's family and friends following Rosalía's instructions. Rosalía and her assistants took the medicinal leaves and carefully placed them on the center of the mattress. Then, Rosalía and her assistants placed the medicinal plants in a column that began on the mattress deposited inside the house and ended in the *rewe*. The *rewe* was located about twenty meters from the entrance door, diagonally, in the courtyard. In this way, Machi Rosalía generated a carpet of leaves, approximately two centimeters thick, from the mattress where the patient would lie to the *rewe*. Red *copihue* flowers (Chilean bellflower) were delicately laid along the carpet of leaves.

The *rewe* itself was also "dressed" in medicinal leaves and red *copihue* flowers.

As there were two machi involved, the ceremony required a specific organization of the space for each machi. Rosalía did not use Ana's *rewe*. Instead, a *rewe* was built for her, where she delivered her message while in trance. Ramón, Rosalía's husband, was the one in charge of building his wife's *rewe*. About ten meters in front of the entrance door to the house, in the *patio* (courtyard), Ramón buried in the ground a branch of *canelo* tree and two flags tied to the tip of *coligüe* sticks. One flag was white and the other one had two horizontal bars, one white and the other one blue. In this way, Ramón designated the place where Rosalía would go into trance, her transitory *rewe*. At the same time, Rosalía took great care in keeping Ana connected to her *rewe* through a carpet of medicinal leaves and flowers. This preparation is aligned with the conventional belief that a machi's spirits are jealous and envious. Therefore, two machi together always carries with it the potential to negatively provoke the spirits. To avoid that, a clear demarcation of space and roles was needed. Each machi needed her own space. If this was done properly, conflict between the spirits of both machi would be avoided.

At 9:30 in the morning the ceremony had not yet started, which was considered by most a significant delay. The reason for the delay was that Ana and her family had not gathered enough branches of native trees to dress the *rewe*. Only after this task was finished did several men take out the old branches of the *rewe* and tie new branches to it. Four native tree species were used: *canelo*, *boldo* (Peumus boldus), *laurel*, and *maqui* (Chilean wineberry). A branch of each species was placed on each side of the *rewe* and tied tightly to it. In addition, new flags were attached to the *rewe*. While the *rewe* was being dressed, several people commented in a reproachful tone about the poor state of it. Some people said that Machi Ana should have renewed her *rewe* some time ago. Machi Rosalía explained that the flags in the *rewe* were important because some machi receive their powers through the flags (that was the case both for her and Ana). Therefore, the fact that Ana's flags were old and neglected was interpreted by some as a transgression. This neglect could explain, at least in part, why the spirit of the machi moved away from her, leaving her powerless.

Machi Rosalía's Trance

To begin the ceremony, Ana lay down on the mattress, her head facing the entrance door to the house (east), while Rosalía sat in the chair by her side. On the house's porch, just in front of where Ana was lying, four *llancan* (ritual dancers), two women and two men, were standing, two for each machi. The male *llancan* held *coligüe* rods with flags on their ends and the women held *canelo* branches. The rest of the participants formed a semicircle at the feet of Machi Ana.

Ramón, Rosalía's husband, played a significant role throughout the ceremony. He was Rosalía's *zugumachife* (ritual interpreter) and was perceived by the audience and Ana as someone who possessed valuable medical knowledge. In fact, he was perceived as having as much knowledge as his wife. It was Ramón who initiated the ceremony by asking Ana's family to ask God for Machi Ana's recovery. One *ngen kutran* or member of the family responsible for the sick one (S: *dueño del enfermo*), should speak on her behalf. Ana's daughter spoke out. People expected Ana's husband to do it because a husband is responsible for his wife's health (a wife is responsible for her husband's health, and parents for their children's). Ana's husband was considered by some of my friends as someone who did not become engaged in his wife's role as a machi. This lack of engagement was judged as a sign of ignorance about the responsibilities of a machi's spouse. He was perceived as someone uninterested in Mapuche practices and knowledge, which could have a negative impact on Machi Ana's health and performance as a machi. The contrast with Machi Rosalía's husband, who was essential to Rosalía's practice as a machi, made the lack of involvement of Ana's husband even more apparent. Ana's daughter started by apologizing because she could not speak Mapudungun. Ramón reassured her by saying: "You'll also be heard in Spanish." She thanked Machi Rosalía and all who were present for being there. She asked for the ritual to be effective and for her mother to recover her health.

The ceremony continued with Rosalía chanting a prayer. She explained that Machi Ana was sick, that she had lost her powers, and asked God to give her back her health and strength. Then, Rosalía started playing her ritual drum. Every time she did this, musicians accompanied her with wind instruments, the rhythmic sound of the *kaskawillas* (a ribbon or leather band tied to the hand to which bronze bells are attached) and the *kultrun* (ritual drum). Several men were holding *wiños* (wooden canes used in the *palin* game or ritual hockey) and hit them against each other to add another sound to the rhythmic and monotonous music.

When the machi resumed her sung prayer, the audience became silent again. This time she chanted while touching the body of the sick machi with two knives. Rosalía firmly pressed the blades of the knives, on the blunt side, over Ana's entire body. Then, Rosalía ingested red wine and spat it out in such a way that a kind of dew of wine fell on the body and head of Ana, as well as over the heads of those closest to her. Rosalía told her husband, Ramón, to give wine to the *pifilkeros* (men playing the *pifüllka or* Mapuche flute). She then began to exhale cigarette smoke on Ana's body. The musicians resumed the music when the machi began again to play her *kultrun*.

After about fifteen minutes the music stopped. Ana seemed agitated and shouted that she had seen Santiago (a friend who was present) approaching her with a small glass containing a yellow *lawen* (medicinal infusion). A man shouted: "*Wezanewen papai*!" (evil energies sister!). Evil spirits usually disguise themselves as someone close, such as a friend or relative, thus nobody thought Santiago had anything to do with the machi's vision. Rather, her vision was immediately interpreted as an indication of the presence of evil spirits. Machi Rosalía responded by saying that we needed more "weapons." Therefore, large kitchen knives and rakes were distributed among the participants. Rosalía also asked for a strainer, which she used to filter a medicinal infusion she had prepared using medicinal plants. Ana's male *llancan* (ritual dancer) gave it to her to drink.

The loud and monotonous music resumed for another fifteen minutes. Then, Rosalía asked the audience if anyone knew how to fire a shotgun. Two men answered positively. These men, one of them Ana's husband, stood in the courtyard, with the main door to the house to their backs, with shotguns in their hands. Machi Rosalía explained to them that they must "walk as if you are looking for something, so you scare the devil" (S: *demonio*). Machi Rosalía also instructed the men to bring the shotgun shells after shooting, so Machi Ana could smell them. This is a counterhex.

The music resumed for the fourth time, which was the last time before Rosalía went into a trance. While the music continued to play, Machi Rosalía, with the help of the two female *llancan*, massaged

Ana vigorously, rubbing leaves of medicinal plants all over her body. When the scrub (S: *friega*) was finished, Rosalía began dancing throughout the house, holding her two knives. Ramón followed her, playing Rosalía's ritual drum, together with other musicians and the *llancan.* The two men holding shotguns outside started shooting, and the noise of the shots, added to the musical instruments, was deafening. Machi Rosalía ran through every room in the house, dancing and pounding her knives, and then ran out the house through the back door. She turned around outside the house to the front yard, followed by her husband, the ritual dancers, the musicians, and some members of the audience. The men who were shooting also followed her, each one firing the gun up into the sky at least five times. The rest of the group remained inside the house with Machi Ana, while some women helped her to get dressed.

The people who stayed inside the house next to Ana were impressed by how fast Rosalía ran. She ran around the yard, around the house, out of the plot's entrance gate, and through the area where potatoes were planted. The people who followed her had difficulty keeping her pace, even though many were young men. She disappeared from our sight and then reappeared unexpectedly, in a different place, on several occasions. When we could not see her, we could still hear the music and the shooting. It was evident for those present that the machi was possessed by her spirit. "She is in trance," a friend told me.

Machi Rosalía returned to the place where Ramón had placed the flags and the canelo branches, about ten meters to the front of the entrance door to the house. Rosalía, Ramón, and Ana sat in chairs in front of the canelo branch and the flags, while the audience was standing behind them. Rosalía, while in trance, played her *kultrun* and delivered a list of remedies and instructions to Ana in the form of a chant. Ramón, performing as her *zugumachife* (ritual interpreter), asked for a piece of paper and a pen to take notes of what the spirits were instructing. The instructions consisted of a long list of medicinal plants to perform a *sahumerio* (incense burning) in Ana's bedroom. Ana was also told she should change the percussion membrane of her ritual drum in a small ceremony, as well as her knives. More remedies were instructed to be used on that occasion. Moreover, the spirits reassured Ana that she was a *küpan* (lineage) machi, thus affirming her legitimacy as a machi. In addition, the spirits said Ana could recover if she followed their advice.

Machi Ana's Trance

After Rosalía delivered a message from her spirit while in trance, the music and the dance were resumed. From that moment on, it was Ana, and no longer Rosalía, who was the leading performer. Ana approached her *rewe* and began to circle around it from left to right. The rounds around the *rewe*, dancing *purrun* (ritual dance), should always be done from right to left. The error did not go unnoticed and generated negative comments during and after the ceremony. Rosalía corrected Ana by taking her by the shoulders and changing the direction in which she was moving.

Despite the mistake made, everyone remained focused on the ceremony. The musicians now accompanied Machi Ana, who danced and played her *kultrun*. The participants encouraged Ana in many ways: with shouts of encouragement and music; pouring spring water and *muday* (fermented wheat) over her head; exhaling cigarette smoke over her body. When the machi began to climb the steps of her *rewe*, great expectation was generated. Climbing the *rewe* was an indication that the machi was in trance. Ana climbed her *rewe* with visible difficulty and required several people to hold her and push her up. This was a concrete manifestation of how weak she was. Despite her evident lack of fitness, Ana managed to stand on the last step of her *rewe* but not at the tip as I have seen other machi doing.

When Ana began to chant while in trance, another uncomfortable moment occurred. There was no *zugumachife*! Rosalía had a worried expression and told her husband, "Nobody is answering her." Ramón began to ask aloud, "Who is going to answer her?" Some people pointed to Jaime, Ana's colleague in the Mapuche medical center. People knew that Jaime was fluent in Mapudungun and performed as a *ngenpin* (master of words, the person in charge of prayers during *ngillatun* rituals) in the *ngillatun* ritual of his *lof* (political territory). Therefore, the audience knew Jaime could perform as a *zugumachife*. Jaime had no other option but to accept the role.

Even though Jaime agreed to be the *zugumachife*, he was worried and angry. Machi Ana had not warned him she was expecting him to perform as *zugumachife*. Therefore, he had not prepared himself properly. That morning, before leaving home, he should have prayed to ask for protection and good fortune. The role of *zugumachife* is tremendously important and mistakes have consequences as serious as those committed by machi. If Jaime made a mistake, both he and his family could become sick. Not to ask Jaime in advance was considered a reckless act on Ana's part. This negligence caused several of the people present to worry about the consequences this could have for Jaime. It also played an important part in the fact that some of the participants strongly disapproved of Ana's performance. Despite the impasse, the ceremony continued without interruption. In fact, not everybody noticed Jaime was an improvised *zugumachife*.

With Jaime now performing as a *zugumachife*, Ana continued chanting and playing her ritual drum while in trance. The machi spirit told the audience that the machi was lonely. The spirit added that the machi could not celebrate *wetrinpantü* (Mapuche New Year) because she did not have enough people to perform the ceremony. At this moment the machi broke down and cried, interrupting her chant momentarily. It happened on two occasions. The audience tried to cheer her up with shouts of encouragement. *Newentulei!* (be strong!)—people shouted.

The fact that Ana cried during trance generated different reactions among those present. For some, it generated feelings of sympathy toward the machi, together with feelings of concern. For others, especially older people who had attended various ceremonies of this type, to cry is a sign of severe illness: it indicated the machi spirit was still disconnected from her. In other words, it showed that the trance was not authentic; that is, the machi was not possessed by her spirit. A friend explained that Ana could have cried at other moments of the ceremony, such as when she was lying on the mattress, or when she was sharing a meal or during the discussions around the *rewe* at the end of every Mapuche ceremony. But to cry while in trance meant that the spirit was crying, and spirits do not cry in such a way. Furthermore, some people think that to cry while in trance is a manifestation of a lack of faith in the *zatun* ritual. The spirits had said, through Machi Rosalía, that Ana, despite being sick, could recover because there were remedies for her. Thus, that Ana cried was a sign that she did not trust the remedies that were given to her. Jaime, visibly upset, told me that Ana had said while in trance that she wanted to die: "My father cried in a *ngillatun* ritual and then he died," he added. Ana did not literally say she wanted to die, but crying was a way of saying she had given up, in Jaime's view.

What Went Wrong?

As in most of the Mapuche ceremonies I observed, people expressed doubts about whether the ritual was being carried out properly. In the ceremony at hand, some of these doubts referred to Machi Rosalía's actions. For instance, some participants were worried about the fact that the ritual was not done twice. As stated above, *zatun* rituals are commonly carried out two times, one at nightfall and then again at dawn. Instead, on this occasion, the ritual was performed only in the morning. In fact, some guests arrived at 6 p.m. When they were told they were supposed to arrive at six, they assumed it was in the evening, because that is the time of day in which a *zatun* ritual usually begins. The guests who arrived late seemed quite puzzled. Another issue that received some commentary was the ritual use of red wine (controversies regarding the use of red wine in traditional ceremonies are further explored in Chapter 5). Some members of the audience judged the use of wine as a transgression of the ritual's protocol. However, others explained that the wine is used to make the *wekufe* (devil) drunk and weak, and to give power to the participants, so they can perform their duties without becoming tired.

The doubts expressed above were not serious enough as to compromise Machi Rosalía's credibility. Serious concerns were centered on Ana, not Rosalía. Critics were centered on Ana for at least two important reasons. Firstly, there is a belief that the sick person is the one who can make more mistakes because she is the weakest, morally and spiritually. In fact, usually, the sick person should remain passive during a *zatun* ritual while other people assume responsibility for the preparations and the performance of the ritual. A friend of mine put it this way: "The sick person is the one to blame, better for him to stay quiet" (S: *el enfermo es el culpable, mejor que se quede calladito*). However, on this occasion, Ana led the second part of the performance, exposing herself to criticism while already being in a weak position. Secondly, the mistakes Rosalía made were subject to controversy, with mixed opinions about them. They were the usual controversies after a ritual performance, which do not seriously affect the perceived efficacy of the ritual. In this way, the machi can provide an explanation as to why the ritual was performed only once. After all, machi are the experts. In this case, Rosalía explained that she had received an instruction from the spirits that the ritual should only be performed once, which was convincing for most people. In the same vein, there are good reasons for using wine in a ceremony and the matter remains an open controversy. Instead, the mistakes Ana made were indisputably mistakes, at least for the people with previous experience of participating in a *zatun* ritual.

Three mistakes generated the strongest concerns, and even anger, among some of the participants. They were serious enough to compromise the perceived authenticity of the machi. The first concern was to not have properly discussed the ceremony with a *zugumachife*. Machi choose a *zugumachife* following spirits' instructions through dreams, visions, and trance. Thus, to randomly select whoever is present only because he can do it is negligent. Moreover, some friends were worried and angry because Jaime was not warned that he was going to perform as *zugumachife*. This omission was interpreted as reckless and dangerous because it put Jaime and his family at risk. It could only mean that the machi was very sick, so sick that maybe she was not going to recover. Some people insinuated that it could also mean that she was never a real machi. It was so hard for them to believe that a machi could forget to talk with her *zugumachife* that people wondered if she ever had the traditional knowledge that every machi needs in the first place. Secondly, people were shocked that the machi circled her *rewe* to the left. Again, this could mean either the extreme severity of her sickness or her lack of *kimün* (ancestral knowledge). Lastly, the fact that Ana cried during trance was perceived by many people as a sign of weakness and extreme severity of sickness. It was a sign that some people interpreted as indicating that her spirit was not there; that is, she was not really in trance. In this way, the deployment of emotions that are considered inappropriate to the ritual context generated doubt about a crucial aspect of the *zatun* ritual; that is, whether the spirit had possessed the machi, talking through her.

Other authors have described how inappropriate performances generate concerns regarding the authenticity of the performers. Frequently, these doubts relate to whether the spirits or gods are in fact present through a medium. Merz (2007) described a healing ritual in which mediums were possessed by gods among the Newars of Nepal. The participants expressed doubts as to whether one of the mediums was possessed: "The doubts related paramountly to the fact that the goddess wept almost uncontrollably, and for a very long time" (ibid.: 218). Schieffelin (1996: 67) wrote that "for Kaluli, the contrast between a good and a bad séance is that between the actual presence of a 'performer' who is consciously trying to deceive them, or in other words, between authentic mediumship … and false pretences …" Thus, an imperfect performance compromises the perceived authenticity of the performer.

There is a normative dimension of ritual activity that has to do with the repetition of actions according to convention. This in an aspect that ritual and custom share: tradition justifies their practice, which is guided by specific rules (Lewis 1980). Conventional rules about how ritual actions should be performed are significant in creating a subjunctive mode and inducing a liminal state in which transformations may occur. In the specific context of rural Mapuche lifeworld, *kimün* (ancestral knowledge) is perceived as a source of shared worth that has been under threat and must be protected and revitalized. Machi play an important role in recovering and transmitting *kimün*. Thus, machi are expected to fulfil a role as depositories of ancestral cultural practices and facilitators of their perpetual repetition by the new generations. Executing actions according to the ritual protocol becomes indispensable for the survival of the ritual itself and, at the same time, for the community that makes it possible. Only through conventional repetition does ritual action allow for the continuing creation and recreation of a ritual congregation. Moreover, ritual claims to be an eternal reality (Seligman et al. 2008: 73–74), which is maintained through the repetition of actions that lead to the same end. Engaging in ritual action is a way of generating a shared sense of belonging to an endless community.

Ana's mistakes, then, are a threat to the continuity and survival of the Mapuche people. This can explain why her mistakes were not ignored and her reputation was damaged, at least in the short term. Rosalía tried to correct the mistakes: she made Ana change the direction of her dance around the *rewe* and, when she realized that there was no *zugumachife*, she made Ramón get one from the audience. There was nothing Rosalía could do about Ana crying during trance. These reparations were not enough to dissipate the strong dissatisfaction with Ana's performance among some of the participants. After the ritual event, I heard for some time reproachful comments about the ritual. These comments reinforced already existent rumors about the machi being a witch. Significantly, these comments reached the ears of people who had not noticed the mistakes during the ceremony because they did not have enough experience of participating in these events.

The Inability to Perform: A Woman Who Cannot Become a Machi

For a healer to be perceived as powerful, or feeble, or fake in giving a diagnosis or treating an illness, they must first perform as a healer. Although this may seem like a triviality, risking a performance is something only some people are willing to try, and not all of them become healers. In fact, most machi tell stories of long and arduous initiation processes. It is not uncommon for people to abandon initiation processes, either permanently or for long periods. These processes usually start with a call from the spirits in the form of varied physical and emotional symptoms, together with financial and interpersonal losses and misfortunes. In order to become a machi, the person who is being called should accept the spirit and learn how to receive knowledge and inspiration from it.

There is a consensus among the machi I met that to become a machi you need to learn and acquire skills. The previous idea does not seem to contradict the, also common, conception that machi receive knowledge and skills through direct inspiration from the spirits. Both statements, although apparently contradictory, are equally true and important in a machi's perception of themself. For example, a machi told me that as a child she knew who was sick and what illness that person had. At the same time, she did not know what to do with these intuitions: how to say what is known, which remedies to use, how to trust your own gut feeling. In fact, all the machi I met told me that they were not able to understand or recognize the call of their spirit at first.

Most *machil* (machi initiate) seek the help of another, more experienced machi to gain the skills and knowledge they need to perform as a healer. Young initiates usually stay at an experienced machi's home for months, observing and assisting their teachers in their role as healers. This interchange usually involves the initiate's family paying the machi in cash. In return, the machi provides food and accommodation, besides teaching. In my observations, these relationships between initiate and machi usually end in quarrels and feelings of betrayal. Thus, it is common for machi to pretend they did not have a teacher; most would say, "I became a machi on my own" (S: *me levanté sola*). It is also common for initiates to change their machi and go to another one after a dispute (or the lack of progress in an initiation process).

Here, I explore an incomplete process of initiation, which allows for the further exploration of performative efficacy in ritual healing. Marta, a machi initiate, believes she is not yet prepared to perform as a healer because she cannot understand the messages she is receiving from the spirits. It was not that Marta could not become a machi because her performances were perceived as unconvincing. Rather, Marta was refusing to perform in the first place. Presenting the material I gathered through a year of conversations and interactions with Marta and some of her friends, I argue that Marta's inability to perform was due to her expectation of being a passive receiver of inspiration coming from the spirits. She had yet to realize that, because the spirits are invisible, a machi should make them visible through imaginative therapeutic techniques. Instead, Marta was expecting the spirits to be visible in the way a bone tumor can be visible in an X-ray. In contrast, skillful machi make the spirits present through healing action, instead of waiting for the spirits to be present before acting.[6] Therefore, if it was not due to the skillful healing actions performed by a machi, the spirits and their inspiration would not be made present.

A Machi Call

Marta was a single mother of two. She was in her early forties and lived with her children in a town near Temuco. She was employed as an "intercultural facilitator" in the local hospital. The fact that she was fluent in Mapudungun and respected among Indigenous communities helped her secure a job in the public health sector as a mediator between Mapuche patients and the medical staff.

There were two elements that made Marta an atypical *machil*. First, her age, given the fact that most *machil* are teenagers or in their early twenties. Second, the fact that she did not live in a rural community, but in an urban area. Mapuche people tend to expect machi to live in rural communities, as it is believed that machi spirits are connected to territory. Despite these atypical characteristics,

Marta was recognized as a machi in a *zatun* ritual, which gave her legitimacy among kin and friends.

Marta had started feeling chronically sick a few years before I met her. Her symptoms began suddenly, were multiple, and continued to change through time. The most debilitating one was an extreme, generalized pain that could get so intense as to impede her from walking. Other symptoms were fatigue, irritability, abdominal pain, and heart palpitations. Marta had gone to several doctors, who carried out multiple tests. Medical tests always showed the same result: "nothing is wrong." According to Marta, the fact that doctors could not explain her symptoms was the first occurrence that made her consider the possibility of a spiritual illness. Furthermore, she started having doubts about whether her affliction was a machi *kutran* (illness), which is understood as a spiritual call from the spirits.

Besides pain and illness, there are other signs indicating a person may be experiencing a machi call. In Marta's case, she realized that even though her family was a Christian evangelical family, who had abandoned Mapuche ritual life, she always felt attracted toward Mapuche practices. Marta told me: "I realized I could speak Mapudungun when I was sixteen. Nobody in my family used to speak the language. I just suddenly realized I was a Mapudungun speaker. I went to several machi, and they all agreed that I have a machi spirit." Marta interpreted her sudden fluency in Mapudungun as a spiritual gift (S: *don*).

When Marta suspected she may have a machi spirit, she went to see several machi, who performed uroscopies and confirmed her suspicions. Initially, she thought she could "buy" the spirit. By this she meant she could pacify the spirit by performing ceremonies in which she should sacrifice an animal as an offering. In this way, the spirit may accept her rejection of the call and find another suitable person in her family to become a machi. However, Marta continued to feel sick to the point of constantly being absent from work. Therefore, she decided to perform a *zatun* ritual so her spirit could tell her what was expected of her.

Marta's *zatun* ritual was presided over by Machi Jorge. It took place about a year before I met her. The purpose of the ceremony was to make Marta's spirit present and receive instructions from it as to what was wanted from Marta. Thus, it was not expected that Marta would start performing as a machi right after it. Rather, the *zatun* ritual was thought of as a confirmation of Marta's machi call, which would finally lead to Marta's complete initiation. On that occasion, Marta went into a trance and her spirit introduced itself. As Marta and other people who participated in the ceremony told me, after the *zatun* ritual was over, most of the participants had no doubt that Marta had a machi spirit. In other words, Marta's performance was perceived as confirming her machi call. The spirit also said Marta needed to learn and train before performing as a machi and that she should receive the support of her family and community. This ceremony was a transformative experience for Marta as she told me that, after it, Mapuche spirituality and ritual life became a central part of her life. She even became, in her own words, "more traditional;" for example, she stopped celebrating Christmas because she considered it alien to the Mapuche, and she started dressing in traditional Mapuche clothing every day. Furthermore, the ceremony involved family and friends, so it was the occasion on which Marta's inner circle became aware of her machi call.

Marta chose Machi Jorge to guide her spiritual initiation after he presided over the *zatun* ritual. However, when I met Marta, she was no longer seeing Jorge regularly. She thought the machi was asking for things that she could not give, such as the involvement of her family and community in her initiation process. Furthermore, the machi's home was far and difficult to access, and the treatment was too expensive. She had to pay 20,000 CLP (US$27) for a uroscopy and medical infusions, but on top of that she had to pay for transport to get to the machi's home. Marta acknowledged that Jorge had said she might be able to become a machi without any help (S: *levantarse sola*). In addition, Machi Jorge had said that another machi, María (a close friend of Marta's), may be better prepared to guide her.

Marta told me about the last time she had seen her machi. She had decided to go to the machi's home because she was feeling very sick. "I took my urine, so he would believe me that I was sick. When he saw the urine, he was dejected and held his head in his hands for a long time. He couldn't believe how sick I was! I told him that my family would not support me." On that occasion, it was decided that Marta should stay at the machi's house to receive remedies and to perform prayers. The night Marta spent at her machi's home she could not sleep at all because evil spirits were bothering her. She kept feeling and seeing dark figures in the night, which constantly woke her up. That the evil spirits were there and her machi could not make them go away was a bad sign. Thus, Marta was having doubts as to whether Jorge was the right machi to initiate her. She could not decide whether she should instead complete her initiation process alone or should ask Machi María to guide her.

It is common for machi to refer patients to another machi when they think they will not be able to improve a condition. Thus, Machi Jorge was expressing his doubts regarding his ability to help Marta when he referred her to Machi María. It is usual for these referrals to occur after long periods of frustrated attempts to recover. In this case, Marta's health was not improving and her ability to perform as a machi had hit a barrier. Also, her commitment to her treatment was erratic, as is shown by the fact that she stopped seeing Jorge for a while. The previous was due to two reasons. Firstly, a practical one: the treatment was expensive and difficult to access. Secondly, Marta was ambivalent toward Jorge and, even though she admired the machi, she had never been convinced that he was the right machi for her.

Marta was not sure about Machi María either. The women were close friends and Marta frequently assisted María when she was presiding over community ceremonies. María was the only person who told me she did not think Marta had a machi spirit, even after attending Marta's *zatun* ritual. The main reason María gave as to why Marta was not really a machi was the fact that spirits do not call people in their forties. Thus, María simply stated that Marta was too old to become a machi. Instead, María thought Marta was a *lawentuchefe* (herbalist) who could treat *rekutran* (common natural diseases) using herbal remedies. But she should not treat spiritual diseases (something reserved for machi). Furthermore, María thought Marta lacked the family and community support necessary to become a machi. Therefore, Marta's doubts about which machi to choose as a teacher were accompanied by the potential teacher's doubts about her chances of becoming a machi. Unfortunately for Marta, her problematic circumstances as a landless single mother, and maybe some rivalry, made it difficult for her to find a committed teacher.

Whether Marta needed guidance in her initiation and who should guide her were not the only doubts she was facing. In addition, she did not have the support of her family and her community. In fact, Marta was the only adult in her household. Usually, *machil* are supported by their families and communities. Important people in a machi's practice, such as a *zugumachife* (ritual interpreter) and other assistants, are family members, such as parents, siblings, aunts, uncles, and spouses. Also, family members usually pay for a young initiate to live with a more experienced machi and for initiation ceremonies. In Marta's case, with two children who were dependent on her, it was just impossible for her to stay with a more experienced machi for a long period of time.

When discussing the lack of support from her family, Marta told me of a dream in which she was on the metro in Santiago. In her dream, she was going to the airport: "That was my spirit searching for my family," she said. In Santiago lived a sister with whom she did not get along and who did not come to her initiation ceremony. Marta believed that the dream indicated that her sister would eventually feel the pressure to visit her. Then, her process of becoming a machi might move faster. But, at the same time, Marta doubted whether her family would ever be willing to become involved. Marta's mother and older brother were deceased. Her father was old and ill. Two siblings living in rural communities had converted to Pentecostalism and, thus, did not participate in Mapuche ritual life. Moreover, her sister who lived in Santiago had not visited her for some time. Machi Jorge said that she could become a machi without the support of her family, but Marta had doubts about whether that could be the case. She expressed that after her *zatun* ritual "everybody abandoned me." Although the participants heard the spirits saying that Marta needed support, once the ceremony was over, she was again on her own.

Landless and without family support, Marta would find it very difficult to become a machi. These are serious practical impediments. However, her own explanation was that the main reason why she could not perform as a healer was her inability to receive direct inspiration from her spirit.

Cloudy Vision and Mysterious Dreams

When I first met Marta, I thought she was a machi. She was assisting another, older machi, in a ceremony. Marta portrayed authority and ancestral knowledge of Mapuche ritual life. She could do things most people cannot, such as speaking fluently in Mapudungun and interpreting the meaning of dreams. Moreover, Marta frequently reprehended people when they committed mistakes in ritual protocols. For instance, she once publicly reprehended a headman because the branches of the *rewe* or altar were not the same height. In addition, she spoke angrily during a ceremony about how outrageous it was because women were not using the traditional Mapuche clothing.

I was not the only one who assumed she was an ancestral authority the moment I met her. In fact, it was common for people to assume Marta was a machi. However, she was visibly uncomfortable when people asked to see her as a machi after assuming she was one. She told me she did not want people to believe she was a machi, not even to know she was in the process of becoming one, because she did not yet feel ready to diagnose and treat. Two things, in Marta's own understanding, were impeding her from completing her initiation. Firstly, that she could not see the urine. When presented with a patient's urine, she could not see anything. "My vision is cloudy, I see everything blurred," she told me. She meant that the actual bottled urine disappeared from her vision and she could only experience anxiety and fear. Secondly, she feared she may not dream before a ceremony. Thus, she would not know what to do. Dreams give information to a machi about what will happen in each ceremony and what she should do. Marta told me: "Dreams tell a machi what she needs to do. In each ceremony, you must act differently, and you know that from the dream. If you do not dream, you will not know what to do. I do not feel ready yet." Therefore, Marta felt she could not do the two most important things machi do: divining and treating through uroscopy and other techniques, and presiding over community ceremonies.

Marta knew that seeing the urine was not only about the sense of vision but also about a direct bodily inspiration or revelation about the patient. Therefore, when she said that her vision becomes cloudy, she also meant that she could not know what was wrong with the patient. Instead, she experienced the fear of making a mistake or performing badly. Marta expected to know the diagnosis without engaging in a reciprocal relationship with the patient. Contrarily, skillful machi direct attention and manipulate emotions to promote the active participation of the patient (as was described in Chapter 2). In a similar vein, Marta expected to know beforehand what was going to happen in a ceremony. She naively expected to know before doing and, thus, refused to perform.

Machi María once tried to encourage Marta to act as a healing person. Marta, María, and I were drinking *mate* tea in Machi María's dining room at nightfall. Marta said she dreamt of her *rewe* (Marta did not have a *rewe* yet, as a *rewe* is built in a machi's home after an initiation process is complete). In her dream, she was in a place that she did not know, a meadow. A soothing male voice she usually heard in her dreams (she told me she thought it was the voice of her spirit) was praying out loud. The prayer was telling her that she was going to receive her *rewe*. In the open field Marta saw her mother, who asked her to serve her a *mate* tea, and her brother lying on the grass (both family members were deceased). She asked her brother to help her, fearing she was not going to be able to hold her *rewe* when it came, so it could fall. Suddenly, she received her *rewe* from the sky in her arms and it smelled like laurel wood. Marta did not have time to see the *rewe* in detail as it had come down from the sky too suddenly. She woke up with her arms open as if she was holding it—she laughed when telling us this.

Before Marta even went through the details of the dream, just after she said she had dreamt of her *rewe*, Machi María exclaimed with excitement: "That's it, you are ready, you are doing what the spirits want you to do! You are already helping people. When people come to you, do what you think you should do." That very same day Marta had brought a colleague who was sick so María could treat him. It was usual for Marta to advise people on health issues, including which machi they should go to. After all, she was working in a hospital and dealing with sick people every day. Thus, María's words were an invitation to action. The words were ambiguous enough to allow Marta a personal interpretation. She could have understood the invitation as the realization that she was meant to be a medicine person but not a machi. But then María said, "When people come to you, do what you think you should do," which is an open invitation to healing action, even the kind of action a machi takes. Marta was not receptive to the machi's words. As usual, she continued to try to understand her dream: does it mean I should use laurel to build my *rewe*? Did my mother also have a machi spirit but did not know about it?

Doubts about how she should act, who she should treat and how, were constant in my conversations with Marta about her dreams.

Even though she was constantly dreaming, she could not figure out the meaning of her dreams. Then, it was not only that she may not dream but also that, even dreaming, she may not know what to do. For example, dreams show a machi the paraphernalia she must use during ritual and medical actions. Thus, in dreams a machi "receives" from the spirits her ritual drum, knives, clothing, and *rewe*. Marta told me: "I dreamed of a white knife that was crooked. Could it be that white should not be the color of my knife? Since it was crooked, I do not know if it means that white should be the color of my knives or not." The impossibility of transforming a dream interpretation into concrete action paralyzed her initiation process. Doubts about the correct interpretation were an obstacle to moving forward. This is also illustrated in the following example. Machi usually play a ritual drum during ceremonies, but Marta was dreaming of another Mapuche instrument, the *trutruka* (a type of trumpet). She could not decide whether this dream was telling her she should play the *trutruka* instead of playing a ritual drum. "The musical instrument that relieves me is the *trutruka*. But I'm not sure if I should play it because it's an instrument that men play. In our culture everyone has their role [gender roles] and that must be respected," said Marta.

Marta also felt insecure about the type of machi she should be. Different machi have different specialties; for example, they treat specific types of afflictions or people, they use specific divinatory techniques, they use specific remedies. Marta shared another dream with me: "I dreamt I was surrounded by children, which could mean that I am supposed to treat children. But it could also mean that I am supposed to guide Mapuche people, who are today like children, because they have lost their *kimün* [ancestral knowledge]." In this way, Marta's dreams, which should be a source of inspiration and action, were, instead, a source of fear of making a mistake.

Within medical anthropology, plenty of attention has been paid to how ambiguity and multiplicity contained in medical diagnosis and illness narratives can promote the exploration of possible explanations and solutions, facilitating action (e.g., Good 1994: 135–65). Following this line of thinking, Marta's doubts could in fact be a driving force causing her to explore multiple possibilities. However, she felt that her situation was stuck and expressed her fears of never being able to become a machi. Thus, it seemed that Marta was not moving forward in her initiation process, neither was she gaining confidence and skills. In other words, she felt paralyzed. The foregoing contrasts with Machi María's excitement upon hearing that Marta had dreamt of her *rewe*. Her words were ambiguous and open-ended, but, contrarily to Marta's doubts, they also contained a push for action, an invitation to transform a cryptic dream into a gift from the spirits.

Marta was not able to make the spirits present through ritual action. Therefore, her refusal to perform as a healer impeded her from receiving inspiration, as Machi María suggested when telling her, "You are ready … do what you think you should do." Instead, Marta thought she lacked inspiration and could not make sense of the spirits' messages. It would be possible to frame Marta's inability to perform as a failure of imagination. As was described in Chapter 1 for the Catholic Charismatics in the US, healers inculcate the capacity to imagine, specifically to experience visual imagery. Moreover, patients learn how to relate to these images in a spontaneous and immediate way or in a way that is not mediated by cognitive elaborations. Thus, non-symbolical relations of meaning (indexical and iconical) are generated once a person becomes habituated to the sociality of a community. In the case of the Catholic Charismatics, the imaginative capacity to spontaneously experience God's presence, through visual imagery and other sensory modalities, was fundamental for the performative efficacy of ritual healing. As God is invisible, he must be made present through imaginative performance so he can become a lived experience. Therefore, Csordas' (1994a) realization that imagination is a mode of self-process through which God and a person's relationship with him is objectified. In the case of Marta, she had still not learned to make the spirits present through imagination, particularly through spontaneous and immediate relations of meaning that are non-symbolic.

Marta's case bears a resemblance to the case of Chini, a Korean shaman who failed to complete her initiation process (Kendall 1996). Chini, like Marta, was expecting to be the passive receiver of the spirits' power. In her initiation ritual, Chini should be possessed by the spirits, who then can give her the power of inspired speech. When Chini remained silent instead of talking, her teacher (or spirit mother), a powerful shaman, angrily yelled at her: "Hey, do you think some spirit would go as far as to move your tongue for you? … I'm struck dumb by her stupidity" (ibid.: 33–34). The teachers insisted that Chini should tell them she is the spirit, how the spirit feels, why it is there, instead of remaining passive and silent. "To feel the spirits and transmit their will and power to others, she [Chini] must be willing to perform for the spirits, to simulate the spirits. From Chini's perspective, the spirits had not matched her expectations … and lacking inspiration, she could not perform" (ibid.: 50).

In conclusion, I have discussed cases of partial failure and obstructing doubts regarding the efficacy of ritual healing. While the case of Ana illustrated an imperfect performance, the case of Marta shows what is needed to be able to perform in the first place. Ana's performance was perceived as inauthentic and, thus, compromised her credibility as a machi. Ana made several procedural mistakes, especially showing an improper emotion while in trance. The fact that she cried while in trance generated doubts regarding the real presence of her sprit. Therefore, the crucial element of a *zatun* ritual was compromised. In the case of Marta, she lacked the knowledge of imaginative doing. In this way, she could not make the spirits present through imaginative performance. Instead, she was passively waiting for inspiration from the spirits. Both cases are inconclusive stories: whether Ana is going to recover her reputation or Marta is going to become a machi remains to be seen. In fact, both cases probably illustrate common experiences among healers: the experience of failing to perform convincingly and the experience of lacking inspiration or knowledge.

Notes

1. The idea of the infallibility of ritual has already been discussed by Evans Pritchard (1976): oracles cannot fail, and when they do they are reinterpreted as non-occurrences of the ritual (or a performance failure).
2. In a similar vein, Humphrey and Laidlaw (1994: 128) observed that: "ritual is prescribed action, you have to get it right, and yet sometimes it seems that so long as you try, so long as you accept the ritual commitment, it is almost impossible to get it wrong."
3. Polit (2007) argues that because the efficacy of a properly performed ritual is not under question, what is at stake in cases of failure is the responsibility of the performers, who can fail. Therefore, "this view of ritual can have severe social consequences for people involved in a ritual that has failed …" (ibid.: 200).
4. A paramedic working at a rural medical post once told me that she was impressed by Machi Ana going there. The paramedic, a non-Indigenous

woman born in Santiago, thought that machi rejected what she called "traditional medicine" (she was referring to biomedicine). "I was surprised to see how humble she is, and she is such a good patient, she doesn't miss an appointment and she takes her medication," the paramedic told me.

5. The *zatun* ritual has been extensively studied elsewhere (e.g., Lenz 1896; Nuñez de Pineda y Bascuñán 1863). For a more recent account see Bacigalupo (2001: 81–87; 2007: 19–23, 73–78).
6. The inextricable relationship between being and doing has been explored elsewhere in performance studies; for example, Schechner (2002) famously argued that the make-believe performances of everyday life, such as gender or professional roles, create the very social reality they enact. In the case of medical performances, Lévi-Strauss' (1963) well-known story on Quesalid, a man who became a shaman to unveil shaman's tricks, and ended up being, or at least believing, he was a powerful shaman, portrays the tangled relationship between being, doing, and believing.

Chapter 5
Mapuche Politics and the *Wetripantü* Ritual

This chapter seeks to ethnographically explore embodied and discursive practices regarding the *wetripantü* ritual or the "Mapuche New Year" and their interaction with the politics of Mapuche identity. Here, I seek to expand the phenomenological gaze, mostly focused on the historical contingency of the present, to the long-term sociopolitical and historical context of the Mapuche in Chile. In this way, the intent is to portray that ritual healing is part of larger political and social processes and, thus, relevant beyond a purely medical domain.

In their well-known article about different epistemological perspectives on the body, Scheper-Hughes and Lock (1987) describe that the body has been understood as an individual body-self in phenomenology (the individual body), as a natural symbol of social relations in structuralism and symbolic anthropology (the social body), and as the object of surveillance and control by the state in Foucauldian approaches (the body politic). Csordas (1999) draws on Scheper-Hughes and Lock when he attempts to relate ritual healing and politics of identity in terms of their interaction at an individual, social, and political level. Similarly, I follow Csordas (ibid.) in ethnographically exploring the way in which the *wetripantü* ritual articulates Mapuche identity at the level of individual transformations, social negotiations within Mapuche society, and cultural representations of Mapuche identity in Chilean public debates.

First, to describe the interaction between *wetripantü* celebrations and Mapuche identity at a political level, I describe the public discourse that Mapuche intellectuals and political activists have built around the *wetripantü* ritual and its political use as a strategy for enhancing difference from the rest of Chilean society. Thus, I examine how the *wetripantü* is portrayed in newspapers, websites, social media, and other public forums. Then, I describe the *wetripantü* celebrations that took place in the house of a machi. The ethnographic description of the ritual event allows me to account for social negotiations regarding alcohol consumption, which, in turn, has implications for the construction of aspects of Mapuche identity, such as masculinity and religiosity. In this way, at a social level, ritual practice allows for negotiations between social actors within Mapuche society regarding what constitutes being Mapuche. Lastly, on an individual level, engaging in ritual practice provides the experiential link between individual transformations and a collective representation of Mapuche identity based on shared dignity and self-worth.

Wetripantü Ritual and Mapuche Identity at a Political Level: The New Year Starts in June!

Wetripantü is a Mapudungun word that means "new sunrise." Some people use the term *Wüñol Tripantü*, which means "the return of the sun." The term *wetripantü* is commonly translated as the "Mapuche New Year" or "New Cycle" and it is understood as such among my interlocutors. *Wetripantü* refers to the observation that, during the month of June, the sun starts moving from the northeast to the southeast until December, when it starts a reverse path from the southeast to the northeast (Pozo and Canio 2014: 108). *Wetripantü* coincides with the winter solstice in the Southern Hemisphere. Besides designating a phenomenon of nature, the word *wetripantü* is used to designate the celebration that takes place at that time of the year. The celebrations usually take place on June 23 and continue until dawn the next day.

People I worked with explained that the *wetripantü* used to be a family celebration. However, it has increasingly become a community celebration rather than a family one within Mapuche rural communities. In addition, it has started to be held in institutional contexts such as hospitals, schools, and police stations. To do so, these institutions invite (and usually pay) a machi to officiate the ceremony.

The open presence of *wetripantü* celebrations in the public sphere contrasts with the celebrations of the *ngillatun* ritual (described in Chapter 2). While the former is promoted and disseminated through the press, advertising posters on the streets and public buildings, and the internet, the latter remains relegated to the intimate sphere of the community and the family. While there are inclusive invitations for everyone to participate in the *wetripantü*, only selected non-Mapuche people will be invited to participate in a *ngillatun*. It seems that while one celebration seeks to be public and create porous identity barriers with Chilean society, the other must remain in a strictly Mapuche context, with an extremely controlled *wingka* (foreign) presence. While what happens in a *ngillatun* is secret and should not be shared with people who did not participate in the ritual, the *wetripantü* celebrations are made publicly visible. While in a *ngillatun* ritual photographs are strictly forbidden, photographs of communities celebrating *wetripantü* circulate freely through the press, social media, and governmental websites.

Political Discourse on *Wetripantü* as Representation of Mapuche Cultural Difference

Political discourse on Mapuche identity is imbedded in broader Indigenous political strategies in Latin America that Hale (2005) has called "neoliberal multiculturalism." Hale (ibid.) points out that politics of cultural recognition that produce and delimit cultural difference have replaced the idiom of *mestizaje* (racial mixture) in nation-building. Indigenous rights to territory, autonomy, and peoplehood are grounded in cultural difference, which requires the political creation of an Indigenous identity through different practices (Hale 1997). Therefore, Hale (ibid.) describes a historical shift in the character of counterhegemonic politics in Latin America, with an emblematic starting point for the occasion of the Columbus Quincentenary in 1992, which generated concerted Indigenous political action throughout the Americas. This historical shift occurred during the 1990s and was one from national-popular movements based mostly on class divisions to political action from marginalized sectors of society, such as women, LGBT groups and

Indigenous peoples. In Chile, neoliberal transformations occurred in the 1980s and were later accompanied by the adoption of multiculturalism with the advent of democracy in the 1990s (Richards 2013). Although "neoliberal multiculturalism" has encouraged Indigenous groups to become citizens and has granted cultural rights, it has also pushed Indigenous communities into highly unequal negotiations for resources and political power (Hale 2005). What is important to highlight is that, despite ongoing power imbalances, multiculturalism has offered new possibilities for negotiation.

Like other Indigenous groups in Latin America, Mapuche activists seek to create a cultural representation of Mapuche identity as radically different to Chileanness. Discursive practices have been developed based on the idea of recovering Mapuche identity, freeing it from derogatory prejudice and reconstructing new meaning around it as a source of self-esteem. It is compelling what the Mapuche journalist, writer, and activist, Pedro Cayuqueo, said in an interview for a national newspaper. The quote below is an attempt to recover a dignified past, in which the Mapuche were not on the margins of society.

> We were not a tribe who walked naked eating blackberries …
>
> The situation a hundred and fifty years ago was very different from the current one. The Mapuche were not the lower class, trampled by those above. Our ancestors were the lords of the economy, they were the aristocracy.
>
> We were defeated militarily, we are not the poor Mapuche … What we have is a war between gentlemen.
>
> (Michelson and Cayuqueo 2017, my translation)

In the political discourse on the *wetripantü* there is an allusion to nature as a source of knowledge and common sense. Therefore, celebrating the New Year in December goes against common sense in the Southern Hemisphere. This extemporality can only occur in a society so colonized by external elements that it does not realize how these colonial elements contradict common sense and easily observable phenomena of nature. The empirical fact in the Southern Hemisphere, I was told many times, is that between the 21st and the 24th of June of each year, the sun is at its furthest point from Earth, undertaking its return until reaching its maximum proximity on December 21st. The *wetripantü* celebrations coincide with the date on which the longest night of the year occurs and mark the beginning of the rainy reason. The coming rain is meant to purify the earth for the renewal of nature and for the beginning of new plantings and harvests.

The incorrect timing of the New Year celebrations is an expression of a history of colonization that deprived Indigenous peoples of their own knowledge of nature (or their own scientific knowledge). This idea is seen in the common statement, both among Mapuche intellectuals and lay people, that their ancestors knew when the New Year began due to their advanced astronomy. Armando Marileo (2008), a *ngenpin* or master of words and a teacher of Mapuche Philosophy at the Catholic University of Temuco, wrote the following:

> The celebration that we hold year after year in the Indigenous world is not a coincidence, nor a light interpretation or only beliefs of the grandparents. Rather, it is the decoding and understanding that they [the grandparents] developed over thousands of years with respect to the norms of nature …
>
> Therefore, the celebration and date that marks the return of life in this hemisphere … is not the property of any culture. Rather, it belongs to all human beings, animals, trees, rivers, birds, who were born and cohabit in this part of the planet.
>
> (Marileo 2008, my translation)

In the same line, Cayuqueo (2011) wrote the following in a press article:

> [A]lthough the Gregorian calendar, which you and I know, that of the santitos, is correct for the Northern Hemisphere, it is at least curious for this part of the globe … another legacy of the European colonizers, like mange and lice … The case is that the Mapuche, privileged observers of nature, established the winter solstice as the end of their fourth annual cycles: Pukemngen, time of rain; Pewüngen, time of blossoms; Walüng, time of abundance; and Rimü, time of rest.
>
> (Cayuqueo 2011, my translation)

As nature is the source of common knowledge among people who share the same geographical space, the reality of *wetripantü*, as a phenomenon of nature, is shared by all inhabitants of the Southern Hemisphere. Therefore, my interlocutors emphasized that other Indigenous people of the continent have similar celebrations, such as the Andean celebration of *Inti Raymi* in Peru and Bolivia. In this way, Mapuche discourse creates a Mapuche identity that is, on the one hand, different and free from external (Chilean, Catholic, European) influence, and, on the other hand, a source of communality with other "peoples of the south," including Chileans. Or we could say that Mapuche scholars and activists are claiming the universality of Mapuche knowledge for all who share the same nature, while at the same time denouncing the inadequacy of the knowledge of the colonizers, which, then, is no longer universal. In this way, Marileo (2008) invited "everyone without distinction to be a participant, and to endorse and initiate the Campaign of Awareness and Visibility of the New Year of the Southern Hemisphere." Cayuqueo (2011) addressed the Chilean public by saying that "deep cultural changes are urgent. In us, to open ourselves to you; and in you, to accept and recognize yourself in us. It could well be that the We Tripantü is a magnificent bridge of communication. These are my wishes in this new year that has just begun." Both public figures, then, conceive *wetripantü* celebrations as emanating from Mapuche knowledge of nature. But since nature is something that is shared by all the inhabitants of a geographical space, it is common or universal knowledge (or at least it is applicable to all living beings "in this part of the planet").

To position *wetripantü* as a source of common understanding in Chilean society is politically relevant. It subverts ideas about *mestizaje* (racial mixture) as the source of Chilean national identity. Instead, *mestizaje* is raised here as a source of misunderstanding, confusion, and lack of identity, while Indigenous knowledge about nature can be a source of authentic understanding and communication.

Moreover, the discourse on *wetripantü* portrays *mestizaje* as a violent, colonial imposition, rather than a mostly peaceful and unproblematic mixing that gave birth to the Chilean nation. My friends stressed that the ancestral celebration of *wetripantü* was deliberately attacked by the colonizers, who imposed the Catholic celebration of Saint John's Eve to disguise it. Although the Mapuche accepted the celebration of Saint John's Eve (they did not have any other choice), many families continued to privately celebrate the ancestral *wetripantü* and never forgot its meaning. In addition, although many people did forget about it, the "authentic" meaning of *wetripantü* can be "recovered." A *longko* I met in the Municipality of Melipeuco told me the following:

> We celebrate the *wetripantü*, we have always celebrated it and we will continue to celebrate it as long as there are Mapuche in this life. We have pleasant memories of the ancestors. Before, it was more exciting [to celebrate *wetripantü*] but now, at least, we have not forgotten, and we continue to celebrate it. I hope there will be people with more enthusiasm. People who will rescue this noble experience of a people [the Mapuche] they [the whites] want to extinguish. We want the lived life of the Mapuche people never to end. So, we celebrate the *wetripantü*.
>
> (Melipeuco 2017, interview)

The Controversy Regarding the Historical Origin of the *Wetripantü* Ritual

In this section, I examine the controversy between, on the one hand, Mapuche political activists and scholars, and, on the other hand, historians and other academics regarding the historical origin of the *wetripantü* ritual. Why and how Mapuche activists dispute the historical origin of *wetripantü* portrays that Mapuche politics both embrace and exceed the state's multicultural politics of delimiting and managing cultural difference. Thus, I intend to problematize the way Mapuche activists engage in politics of identity.

While historians claim that the *wetripantü* ritual is a recent innovation, introduced in the 1990s, in the context of national and continental Indigenous protests and politics of state cultural recognition of Indigenous identities, Mapuche activists claim that the *wetripantü* ritual has an ancestral origin and derives from Mapuche knowledge of nature or Mapuche scientific knowledge. Defining the timing of the New Year becomes a heated political debate: it is a struggle to define truth by affirming that Mapuche knowledge is both scientifically and historically valid. Thus, the intent is to claim that, despite the common assumption that both history and science are exclusively Western or at least based on Western rationality, Mapuche knowledge is historical and scientific. This is in line with recent political and scholarly struggles to pluralize both history and science.

Some social scientists have questioned the authenticity of Mapuche practices by understanding tradition mainly as a reaction ("invention") to broader social and political phenomena. Since Hobsbawn and Ranger's (1983) influential *The Invention of Tradition*, it is assumed that there are certain practices that are genuinely old, and others that are relatively recent and should be understood as political resistance, reaction, or adaptation. This approach has been influential in the study of Indigenous movements in Latin America (e.g., Briones 2003; Rappaport 1994) and Chile (e.g., Bengoa 2012). Within this framework, Briones (2003:v38) proposed to understand *wetripantü* as a "holy icon," borrowing Hobsbawn's term. Briones described how *wetripantü* was born, among the Mapuche of Argentina, in a meeting held on May 24 and 25, 1991, in Junín de los Andes. According to Briones, on that occasion young political activists were eager to establish the 24th of June as the threshold for the New Year. Contrarily, the elders "marked June 24th as the moment when daylight certainly starts growing at the pace of a cock footprint by day. Still, most of the elders maintained that mid- September marked the proper beginning of the year" (ibid.: 38–39). Briones understands the insistence of young activists on establishing the 24th as the beginning of the New Year, as a strategy of differentiation from Argentinian society, which celebrates New Year in December. In addition, it is a strategy to generate commonality with the Mapuche of Chile and other Indigenous groups of South America, who also celebrate the New Year on the 24th of June. Bengoa (2012), one of the most influential Chilean historians of the Mapuche, claims that, while the *ngillatun* ritual is an ancient practice that can be traced back to colonial chronicles, the *wetripantü* ritual has no clear historiographic record and may have never existed before. Bengoa wrote that Saint John's Eve, a product of hundreds of years of cultural syncretism, has become the *wetripantü*. The historian adds that he thinks the *wetripantu* celebrations in Chile started in the 1990s in Temuco, when a group of Mapuche university students decided to celebrate *wetripantü*. Like Briones, Bengoa understands this process as one of identity reaffirmation and rupture from the *mestizaje* idiom as national identity.

However, my Mapuche friends followed Mapuche intellectuals, political activists, and religious leaders (including machi) in opposing the above academic historians' position. Thus, my interlocutors insisted that *wetripantü* celebrations were practiced before the Mapuche were colonized, and derived from a rigorous observation of nature. Mapuche activists oppose the historians' position by advancing the claim that oral history, lived traditions, and linguistic knowledge constitute proof of the ancestral origin of *wetripantü* and its relation to astronomical knowledge. In this way, they demand state recognition of Mapuche knowledge through the recognition of the historical authenticity of *wetripantü*. Pozo and Canio's (2014) work regarding the Mapuche understanding of the cosmos and astronomy is an example of such an attempt, and one that my interlocutors considered enthusiastically as a way of recovering *kimün* (ancestral knowledge). The authors conducted ethnographic work and interviews with Mapuche rural communities in the Chilean regions of Bío-Bío and Araucanía and in the Argentine Patagonia. The book describes how Mapuche people relate the movement of different stars, such as the *küyen* (moon), the *wüñellfe* (morning star or Venus), the *wanglen* (constellations), and the *antü* (sun), with social activities, such as rituals and agriculture, and also with mythical and historical narratives and traditional songs in Mapudungun. This is what an old man told the ethnographers:

> Aforetime, the Mapuche made a *ngillatun* for the day of the *wetripantü*. So, *Ngenechen* (God) left us the sun, that's why the sun is alive, it is alive, it has life, a lot of life, and the sun is the one we make the *ngillatun* for, we dance for the sun. Is that why the sun is happy? Is that why the sun dances when it just rises? In the old days, people prepared to do a *ngillatun* when the sun was just rising. Before it [the sun] appeared, they prepared the *ngillatun* ... Is that why the sun is happy?
>
> (Pozo and Canio 2014: 110, my translation)

For my interlocutors, the specificity of the Mapuche knowledge about the movement of the stars in the sky and its relationship with the oral tradition on the *wetripantü*, as described in Pozo and Canio's (2014) work, constitutes proof of the historical origin of the ritual. For Pozo and Canio (ibid.), oral traditions and astronomical knowledge constitute evidence of the importance of the sun as a deity in Mapuche cosmogony, which, in turn, confirms the precolonial origin of the *wetripantü* ritual. In this way, Mapuche politics embrace multiculturalism's proposed plurality by struggling to pluralize historical and scientific knowledge.

However, there are other ways in which Mapuche people claim to know the ancestral origin of *wetripantü*. When my friends referred to the Mapuche *kimün* (ancestral knowledge), they thought of it as something usurped that needed to be recovered. Thus, the *kimün* was, in general, something that was missing. However, there were concrete practices through which one could recover *kimün*: ritual performance, dreams, the wisdom of ancestral authorities, such as machi and *longko*, and the content of the Mapuche language. Contemporary Mapuche should know their history as a people not through the reading of academic books and Spanish colonial chronicles. Rather, *kimün* should be accessed through the content of the Mapuche language, which has survived colonization, and dreams and ritual trance, which allow them to be in continuous contact with the ancestors and spirits.

In this way, Mapuche knowledge is not supposed to be read in Western books but acquired through practices in the present, which involve dreaming, participating in ritual events, and talking to the elders and wise people. Mapuche understanding of the past is a dynamic one that involves the constant enactment of the past in the present through language and ritual practice.[1] Therefore, the past should be accessed through action in the present. That is to say that the past is not a static reality left in historiographic record. Rather, through ritual performance, dreaming, and speaking and listening in Mapudungun, the past is susceptible to becoming a present action. Put another way, one could say that for my interlocutors the past is not supposed to be discovered but lived as a present-day experience.

Ahistorical entities, such as spirits and ancestors, participate in the performance of Mapuche past through visions, dreams, and ritual trance. This is a struggle to know the past in Mapuche terms. Here, what is at stake is not the question of the historical authenticity of tradition. Rather, what matters is the spiritual ability of machi to communicate with the spiritual world, which, in turn, constitutes the Mapuche way of knowing the past and the present. Thus, Mapuche activists not only seek the recognition of *wetripantü* as an authentic historical practice, but also as a worlding practice, which enacts a Mapuche world ontologically different to Chileanness. In this way, my Mapuche friends claim an ontologically distinct past that cannot be possible according to historians. Rather, the past enacted through relationships with spirits and ancestors is disqualified as politically irrelevant: unreal or cultural beliefs. History, then, enacts the political act of determining the real. As Marisol de la Cadena (2015: 13) stated: "the historical ontology of modern knowledge both enables its own questions, answers, and understandings and disables as unnecessary or unreal the questions, answers, and understandings that fall outside of its purview or are excessive to it."

Mapucheness here emerges as radically different to Chileanness. However, because this is a historical ontological difference, it cannot be understood as something that the Mapuche possess. Rather, Mapucheness exists in a relationship with Chileanness. This relationship between Mapucheness and Chileanness has been defined as a "partial connection" (De la Cadena 2015: 32–33), meaning that both entities emerge from their historical relation and are, thus, intra-related, instead of inter-related. Therefore, Chileanness and Mapucheness cannot be divided into parts or wholes (ibid.: 32): their relationship is integral and not external to the parts. As De la Cadena (ibid.), drawing on Haraway (1991: 81), and against the multicultural idea that the alternative to one is many, would put it: Mapucheness and Chileanness are more than one and less than many: "Borders between indigenous things and nation-sate things are complex; they historically exist as relations among the fields they separate, and therefore they also enact a connection from which both – things indigenous and non-indigenous – emerge, even as they maintain differences vis-à- vis each other" (De la Cadena 2015: 33).

The idea of Mapucheness existing in partial connection with Chileanness is useful in understanding why Mapuche scholars and activists not only claim their own ontological past (or the past in their own Mapuche terms) but also challenge historians in historical terms. To only emphasize incommensurability between different ontological worlds would be politically unproductive, and Mapuche activists clearly understand what the state can and cannot recognize. Therefore, Mapuche politics exceed, while at the same time embrace and allow multicultural politics of state recognition of cultural plurality.

To summarize, in this section I have addressed the interaction between *wetripantü* celebrations and Mapuche identity at the level of representational practices. Mapuche identity is represented as possessing its own specificity and is, thus, different to the dominant Chilean society. The time at which to celebrate the New Year becomes a heated political issue due to underlying power struggles for knowledge (scientific and historical), tradition and authenticity. Cultural difference is a source of pride and self-esteem, as well as a terrain for political negotiations within a form of governance through cultural recognition.

Wetripantü Ritual and Mapuche Identity at a Social Level: Negotiations on Alcohol Consumption

In this section, I explore how alcohol consumption is negotiated in the course of a *wetripantü* ritual event and how these negotiations are grounded in conflicting social relations within Mapuche society.[2] Thus, I move from the representation of Mapuche identity at a macropolitical level to local negotiations between conflicting Mapuche social actors. Identity at a social level, then, is not only about creating cultural difference from a dominant society, but it also supposes power and moral negotiations within Mapuche communities. In the case at hand, ritual action allows for negotiations regarding what constitutes proper behavior in the context of Mapuche ritual life, which, in turn, has implications regarding the kind of Mapuche masculinity and Mapuche spirituality considered socially desirable.

Mapuche political identity at a social level no longer appears uniform as it did in the previous section. Rather, aspects of Mapuche identity, related to masculinity and religiosity, are negotiated through ritual healing action, which amplifies the complexity of what constitutes being Mapuche. When, how, and if Mapuche men should consume alcohol is the vehicle to negotiate what constitutes proper Mapuche masculinity and religiosity. These negotiations take up themes addressed in the previous section: the creation of a Mapuche identity that is free from derogatory prejudice and a source of pride and self-esteem.

The discussion in this section is mostly based on participant observation during one *wetripantü* celebration at the home of Machi Juana and later informal conversations about the occasion. An important characteristic of the event described here is that this celebration was a healing ritual. It was a healing ritual not only due to the presence of the machi, but for the objectives that, according to the participants, the celebration sought. These objectives were the renewal of the healing abilities of the machi through the renovation of her *rewe* (altar), so she could continue to treat her patients.

In addition, those who participated in the ritual, together with the machi and her community, were the machi's patients, who participated as a sign of gratitude. A woman told me: "We are here because we have been healed by the machi. So, we are here to show we are grateful because of what she did for us. Also, we are here to help the machi to renew her strength and her *rewe*" (Araucanía 2017, interview).

The ceremony began on Friday June 23 at around 1 p.m. and ended on Saturday afternoon at around 3 p.m. The guests arrived little by little throughout the day on Friday and at nightfall (around 6 p.m. at this time of the year) there were about seventy to eighty people at the machi's home. On Friday night, people danced *purun* (ritual dance) for hours around the *rewe* (altar) and inside the machi's *ruka* (traditional house) around the fire. A little after midnight, people dispersed into small groups. Some went to sleep in the machi's house or those of other people in the community who were hosting guests in their homes. Other people remained in the *ruka* or in the dining room of the machi's house, chatting and sharing food. Several stayed awake all night. Some people accompanied the machi and the musicians who periodically danced *purun* around the *rewe*.

The next morning, at 6 a.m., people were called to gather around the *rewe* and they engaged in ritual dancing for about nine hours, with small breaks in between. At dawn, when the dance started, it was cold, dark, and wet. The dance was, little by little, generating expectation as the participants waited anxiously for the message that the spirit would deliver during ritual trance. The message delivered by the spirit promoted a discussion about alcohol consumption that began that same day and continued for some time after the event. Moreover, the message given by the spirit was effective in promoting discussions about a topic that was usually met with resistance in everyday situations. When the machi went into trance, her spirit said that many people were sick. Many were experiencing insomnia and severe headaches. Some of them were sick because of alcohol consumption, the spirit said. The men, including the *longko*, who had gone to gather the branches of native trees to dress the *rewe* the day before the celebrations began, had drunk alcohol when performing this ritual task. This was a grave mistake! The *longko* was especially responsible and he was warned by the spirit that he could become severely sick. To cure people from these disorders, the machi was going to make a burning incense (S: *sahumerio*) with medicinal plants. Everybody who was suffering from headaches and insomnia should come closer to the smoke produced by the medicinal burning incense.

As promised in the spirit's message, the machi, still in trance, grabbed a large metal brazier containing burning fresh medicinal leaves previously collected in the fields. She started running among the bodies of the participants holding the brazier, which looked very light in her hands. Many people commented on how amazed they were because the brazier was, in fact, very heavy. As the machi ran between the participants with the brazier in her hands, hot coals fell to the ground, and she, who was running barefoot, stepped on them. Her feet were not burned, and again people expressed feelings of amazement because she was not burned. This was not the only moment of amazement during the celebration. In fact, it was a celebration full of moments that the participants considered to be extraordinary and that were interpreted as an indication of the genuine connection with the spiritual world. For example, the machi repeatedly stepped on embers without being burned, many sick people felt significantly better during and at the end of the ceremony, and in the moment of ritual trance it started to rain. The spirit explained to the assistants that the rain was sent to purify the earth and the people in this *wetripantü* so that life could continue. During the moment in which the machi was running holding the brazier, we all observed a huge flare of smoke that many people described as being like the eruption of a volcano. All the participants were engulfed by the smoke, and it was difficult to see. A man said that they were receiving the volcano's energy and strength (M: *zegiñ newen*). Moreover, the volcano's ashes were meant to purify their bodies and the land in which they live, driving sickness, misfortunes, and injustices away. Many of my friends told me that when a volcano erupts, Earth is protecting itself from destructive forces, usually derived from human transgressions (such as cutting down the native forest). Therefore, a volcanic eruption is an indication of the strength of Earth to maintain and recreate life.

The extraordinary ways described above in which the spirits communicated with the participants of this *wetripantü* celebration, points to the capacity of ritual performance to create a reality somehow separated from everyday routine. That is to say that the spectacular actions that were carried out, such as stepping on burning coals or holding a heavy metal brazier as if it was light, together with intense emotions, such as amazement, carved a ritual space and time separated from everyday reality. As discussed in Chapter 1, Kapferer (2004) called "the virtuality of ritual" that ritual characteristic that involves the creation of an "imaginal space," where people can reorient themselves to the world and others, and a "technical space," distant from the everyday routine, in which people can actively transform the structures of reality. In this case, ritual action makes possible negotiations on alcohol consumption between social actors who are unequal; that is, women and men, through momentarily altering structural inequalities. Significantly, the leading figure in this ritual event was a woman, and that had tremendous significance in influencing the kind of negotiations that took place. Therefore, through ritual practice, negotiations can occur that are difficult to carry out in the context of everyday micropolitical power negotiations (I discuss gender negotiations further later).

A second message was delivered from the spirit in this *wetripantü* celebration. On this second occasion, the spirit told the audience that the burning incense had exerted its effects and that they were going to feel better soon. The spirit continued by saying that after the ceremony they were going to drink a medicinal herbal infusion (M: *lawen*) that the machi had prepared. This herbal infusion contained hot red wine together with numerous medicinal herbs. The fact that it contained wine was not mentioned by the sprit during ritual trance. However, red wine was easily identifiable when drinking the medicinal infusion, which tasted like mulled wine. In fact, the machi later explained to all the participants what the infusion was for (and she had also talked about it before the ceremony when she and her community were preparing for it). "The spirit wants to teach us how to drink wine," the machi said. I will come back to what it means to know how to drink wine later.

At the end of the ceremony, as is usual in Mapuche rituals, people stayed around the *rewe* to discuss what the spirit had said. By that time, the sun had come out and the temperature had increased significantly. Because the spirit had reprimanded him, the *longko* had to admit that he had drunk *aguardiente* (a grape distillate) when he had left the day before to gather native trees branches to dress the *rewe*. The *longko* was visibly embarrassed. After he apologized to all the participants, other middle-aged men (many had also been drinking with the *longko* the day before) took advantage of the occasion to address young men and tell them that alcohol is "a trap introduced by the *wingka*" (the whites) to muddy and weaken them. Therefore, men should be able to resist the temptation to drink, especially when they are performing their ceremonies. Before the arrival of the *wingka*, the Mapuche did not produce wine or other foreign alcoholic beverages, only *muday* (a beverage obtained from the fermentation of grains of corn or wheat that contains a very low degree of alcohol). The introduction of wine by the Spaniards and its later use by the Chilean Army, severely contributed to the degradation of Mapuche warriors and men in general, said a middle-aged man. Therefore, the recovery of Mapuche practices and identity should include the realization of how foreign practices, such as alcohol consumption, had weakened and depraved them as a people.

Gender Negotiations on Alcohol Consumption

On the occasion described above, it became clear to me that my male friends shared feelings of shame and humiliation. These feelings not only affected the men who had actually been caught drinking, but most of the male participants. To understand these feelings of humiliation and shame and the way some Mapuche men negotiate how, when, and if they should consume alcohol, I will address the historical and social meaning of alcohol consumption among the Mapuche in the Chilean context.

Cornelio Saavedra, the leader of the Chilean Army during the military occupation of Araucanía (1861–1883), famously argued that to win the war was going to take "a lot of alcohol and music, and little gunpowder" (S: *mucho mosto, mucha música y poca pólvora*) (cited from Richards 2013: 39).[3] In this way, the general was trying to convince authorities in Santiago that it was going to be easy to subdue Mapuche political and military leaders because of their proclivity to alcohol and partying. Qualifying the Mapuche as drunks and lazy is a frequent form of insult to this day. In a press article, Chilean historian Sergio Villalobos (2000) proclaimed Mapuche males' tendency to alcoholism as a factor demonstrating the Mapuche cultural backwardness in comparison to the Spanish *conquistadores*.

Villalobos continued to say that it is a universal occurrence that a "more evolved culture imposes itself on a less evolved one."[4]

Although most of the people who comment in public forums today avoid obvious racist expressions such as Villalobos', the historian is far from being the only one using these prejudices to insult a people in a very open way. For instance, the well-known Chilean painter, Carmen Aldunate, published on her Facebook account that Mapuche were "murderers, cowards, lazy and thieves; besides drunks and opportunists." After publishing this post, in an interview about her writings (Améstica and Aldunate 2013), she recognized it was "a mistake to generalize." She explained that she had written the previous statement in a moment of anger after a serious crime, allegedly committed by Mapuche activists, occurred. However, she could not miss the opportunity to devalue the Mapuche again: "Of all the cultures, of all the ethnic groups, the Mapuche, when it comes to the pictorial arts are the poorest. Very primitive. We cannot compare them with Peru or Colombia" (ibid.). Both Villalobos and Aldunate allude to excessive alcohol consumption among Mapuche men to devalue and insult an entire people.

Declarations like that of Villalobos are both a struggle for a hegemonic national identity, based on the process of racial mixture (S: *mestizaje*) as overcoming Indigenous primitivism, as well as a hegemonic masculinity. Two main imaginaries of Mapuche masculinity have been portrayed in Chile's cultural production (Crow 2014). First, the image of the brave Araucanian warrior who defeated the Spanish *conquistadores* during colonial times. This image is contraposed to a second one: that of the Mapuche men today, who are portrayed as lacking self-control and morality (i.e., uncivilized). Behaviorally, Mapuche men's backwardness is expressed through alcoholism and violence. Bacigalupo (2007) has argued that, on some occasions, Mapuche men have appropriated the image of the brave and virile Araucanian warrior to become part of hegemonic masculinity and hegemonic patriarchal national identity. For instance, male machi have tried to conform to normative ideas about masculinity through the identification with warriors, priests, and doctors (ibid.). It appears, then, that what is at stake here is a dignified Mapuche masculinity.

Villalobo's (1995) version of Arauco War (1536–1772), the war between the Mapuche and the Spanish *conquistadores*, is one in which the historian dismisses the intensity of the war and, with it, the courage of the Mapuche warrior. For Villalobos, the Arauco War is a myth in the sense that it is historically untrue. Thus, Villalobos questions the historical veracity of the noble Araucanian warrior. As an alternative, Villalobos proposes that the Araucanians were simply absorbed by a "more evolved culture," the Spanish one, in the slow, mostly peaceful, and inevitable process of *mestizaje*. Cayuqueo's (2017) recent book *Secret Mapuche History* is an attempt to historically demonstrate that the Mapuche counted not only with impressive warriors, but also with statesmen who negotiated with the Chilean and Argentine republics during the nineteenth century and early twentieth century. Interestingly, Cayuqueo put the emphasis not on a glorious past during the Arauco War 500 years ago, but on a more recent past only 150 years ago. This is again a rupture from *mestizaje* as core to the foundation of the Chilean Republic. Rather, Cayuqueo writes about violence, murder, and atrocities committed against the Mapuche and Mapuche efforts to resist colonization in a near past. In Cayuqueo's own words, he is trying to reconstruct a Mapuche history that repairs the damaged self-esteem of his people. In a recent interview for a national newspaper, Cayuqueo expressed the following:

> We are a defeated, humiliated, and despised people and we are just recovering our self-esteem. When black pride arose in the United States, something appeared that for any revindication is very important: human self-esteem. And that [self-esteem] gives you a cultural ethos, a way of seeing the world. And when your way of seeing the world is constantly humiliated, mistreated, you will be sick. We are in the process of healing due to mistreatment.
>
> (Michelson and Cayuqueo 2017)

But what Cayuqueo portrays as Mapuche self- esteem, I consider to be a "male" Mapuche self- esteem.[5] That is to say, that the kind of dignified Mapuche identity Cayuqueo is reconstructing is a masculine one, identified with the past glory of statesmen and male political and economic leaders. Cayuqueo's "male" Mapuche self-esteem resonates with that of my interlocutors. Many of my male friends expressed to me feelings of humiliation because of their situation within the margins of Chilean society. Rural Mapuche men tell stories about experiences of humiliation in the public sphere such as schools, the workplace, and the army. These experiences of humiliation arise both from their ethnic (Mapuche) and social (lower-class) identities. One of my friends, a rural teacher, told me that to know that the Europeans and Chileans who conquered his people were "low-class Europeans," probably "fugitives from justice, and ignorant people," was even more humiliating. For my friend to think that his ancestors, who were *longko*, had to negotiate with people of low status was a source of deep humiliation.

For some of my male friends, the introduction of alcohol by the Spanish and then by the Chileans was a deliberate action to weaken them. Unfortunately, many Mapuche men succumbed to the temptation of alcohol, abandoning their families and social obligations. The poverty of the current rural world is due, at least in part, to that abandonment, I was told by some people. Domestic violence toward women and children, which most men recognize as undesirable and as a problem, is also a product of the moral degradation of men due to the consumption of alcohol. Moreover, some of my friends thought that the reason why spirits stopped choosing males to become machi was, again, due to their moral transgressions, such as alcohol consumption and, significantly, betrayal in their negotiations with the invaders. In the same way, the reason why machi (mostly females) were today more powerful than *longko* (almost exclusively males) was, again, the weakening of the *longko*'s strength due to past moral and spiritual transgressions. The previous ideas, although mainly expressed by men, were shared by many of my female friends, who expressed nostalgia for the times when the *longko* (and the men) were strong.

Returning to the *wetripantü* celebrations at Machi Carmen's house, the issue of men consuming alcohol was a terrain of dispute and tension. As I have already described, the spirit, during trance, reprehended the men and the *longko* who had been drinking the day before while performing a ritual duty. What had happened was that the machi had given the men a couple of bottles of *aguardiente* (a grape distillate). She had done it because, before going to the fields to cut native tree branches to dress the *rewe*, the men should perform a prayer and spread *aguardiente* as a counterhex. When the men came back to Machi Carmen's home, they smelled of alcohol and seemed drunk. I was there with the women when this happened. What the women feared, when they realized the men were drunk, was that they were going to fail in their tasks. Without the men, the ceremony could not be carried out. Thus, the women were nervous and angry. They did not confront the men directly and simply just hoped they would continue to perform their tasks, which they did.

During the ceremony, men were exposed by the message of the spirit. Because of this exposure, men were forced to recognized their mistake. When the error committed by the men was discussed, they used a narrative that I already knew well. The men narrated a historical connection between excessive alcohol consumption, as a current problem, and the common history of dispossession and colonization. In this way, alcohol had been deliberately introduced to humiliate and defeat them. Alcohol is foreign to the Mapuche, it is an evil that comes from outside. They must resist alcohol, just as they must resist all forms of domination. Thus, the discussion went on to focus on a common history of abuse and mistreatment.

Significantly, the women did not speak publicly about this issue in the *wetripantü* celebration described above. To understand the women's perspective, I had to talk to several of my female friends in private. The women's view had different nuances to those of the males. The element that clearly came to the forefront and that had been absent from the men's discussion was domestic violence. That is, women associated alcohol with violence and failure to perform duties toward the family.

Although women did not contradict the idea of alcohol as something imposed from the outside, they introduced a new element when explaining the violence of men; namely, the asymmetry of power between men and women. In this way, women believed that violence against them had originated from the inability of men to value women. Women thought some men considered their wives their property. Women also complained about irrational jealousy and excessive possessiveness. In the women's narrative, the emphasis was placed not on violence perpetrated from the outside by the invaders, but on the violence of intimate relationships perpetrated by fathers, husbands, and partners (also mothers, and in the case of elderly women, sons).

The celebration of *wetripantü* was an opportunity for women to express, indirectly, their discomfort and concern about alcohol consumption. The men were forced to respond and admit their mistake. On other occasions, I witnessed women trying to confront men in their families directly. What usually happened was that men would laugh and start telling funny anecdotes about the behavior of friends and relatives when drunk. This avoidance strategy was usually effective in dismissing the gravity of the problem and preventing any possible negotiation or meaningful discussion. When I tried to talk with some male friends about alcoholism and violence, their attitude was tremendously defensive. The ritual occasion allowed for men and women to agree that both the consumption of alcohol and violent and irresponsible behavior were not acceptable. Thus, they could work together in carrying out the *wetripantü*, which required the segregated labor of men and women. While the women made the bread and the *sopaipillas* (fried bread), gathered medicinal leaves, and prepared much of the ritual paraphernalia, men slaughtered the animals, drove the vehicles to bring goods and people, and gathered big branches of trees to dress the *rewe*.

The hot red wine medicine that was announced during trance and later distributed to all the participants was a remedy that was given (S: *entregado*) to Machi Carmen by her spirit in dreams. The machi dreamt of the *wetripantü* celebration and, in her dream, people were drinking wine. She was perplexed at the beginning because, in her mind, wine has nothing to do with a traditional Mapuche ceremony. Thus, she initially thought the dream was a warning that people were drinking wine when conducting ceremonies and that they may be punished because of it. Then, the machi told us, she continued to dream of people drinking hot wine during the *wetripantü*, only this time the wine also contained various medicinal herbs that were, again, given to her in her dreams. When discussing these dreams, as the machi and her community were preparing for the *wetripantü* celebrations, the machi explained that her spirit wanted to "teach people how to drink wine." The machi said that her spirit wanted her to distribute hot wine with medicinal herbs to her guests. In this way, nobody was going to get drunk, because the wine would have been previously boiled, and they were all going to receive medicines. When I asked her what would constitute "knowing how to drink wine," she said that it was fine to drink moderately for social occasions. The problem was the spiritual and moral transgression that drinking supposes if it is done while conducting a religious ceremony. When she said this, the machi was seated at her dining table with several people from her community, who had gathered to prepare the *wetripantü* celebrations. Other people also responded to my question, adding more examples in which drinking was wrong.

Women emphasized violent behavior and men spending all their salary on alcohol. People also mentioned reckless behavior such as driving while drunk or engaging in drunken fights. They also mentioned that it was important not to give the young a "bad example." Therefore, children and young people should not see adults drunk.

Religious Negotiations on Alcohol Consumption

During the *wetripantü* celebration at Machi Carmen's house, some people said that they were angry at the *longko* and the men who had drunk alcohol while performing a ritual duty. Some people thought that they should prove to others that Mapuche ceremonies are not simply "an excuse to get drunk." People were particularly worried about what their Pentecostal relatives and neighbors might say if they found out. Pentecostal Christians mock the Mapuche ceremonies because they consider them simply a social meeting to drink alcohol without control, rather than genuinely traditional practices with spiritual meaning. "That's why Christians are saying that the Mapuche are all drunks," a male friend expressed with some irritation when discussing the issue that some men had been drinking while preparing for the *wetripantü*. In this way, people thought that alcohol consumption while conducting a Mapuche traditional ceremony devoided the ceremony of its religiosity or sacred aspects, transforming it into any ordinary social event. As many people feared more people may convert to Pentecostalism and abandon Mapuche ritual life, the religious or sacred nature of the *wetripantü* celebration was very important to them. "To be Mapuche is to have a religion. We have our own religion," a *longko* told me.

The vehement and persistent condemnation of alcohol by rural Pentecostal Mapuche is a significant source of conflict. For instance, I was present at a funeral in which five brothers buried their mother. Three of the brothers were Christians,[6] while the other two wanted a traditional Mapuche ceremony and had invited the machi and *longko* of their community to perform it. Traditionally, Mapuche people drink wine around the deceased while conversing about the deceased's life. The "Christian" brothers and their families left the place as soon as people started drinking wine. Moreover, when the machi and the *longko* conducted a prayer in Mapudungun while dancing around their diseased mother, the Christian brothers and their families remained at a distance, physically performing the family's internal rupture. I also observed that when Christians refused to drink on social occasions, such as family meetings, christenings, social gatherings among co-workers, or weddings, some people, especially men (but not only), reacted with irritation. "Alcohol is good in small amounts, we don't need to stop drinking," a man said as he confronted a friend who was refusing a drink.

Some of my friends used to categorize the rural Mapuche world into at least three types of people. One group is the Mapuche; that is, people who actively participate in Mapuche ritual life. The second group corresponds to the *awingkados* (Westernized), which refers to Mapuche people who have little participation in Mapuche ritual life and who mostly identify with Chilean society. A third group corresponds to "Christians" (Pentecostal Christians). My friends, most of them more or less Mapuche, consider the group of Christians as antagonists. "Christians" demonize Mapuche religious practices and consider machi to be witches. Converted "Christians" not only abandon Mapuche religiosity, but also family and social ties. As the Mapuche themselves are converted, Pentecostalism constitutes an internal threat to the continuity of Mapuche spirituality and ritual life. My friends explained the high rate of Mapuche converting to Pentecostalism as a new colonizing onslaught. They thought the new missionaries took advantage of the Mapuche's natural disposition to religiosity.

The strong presence of the Pentecostal movement, which vehemently condemns alcohol consumption, has contributed to many people rejecting the presence of alcohol in traditional ceremonies. In this way, people try to avoid accusations that Mapuche ceremonies are simply "an excuse to get drunk." I witnessed, on various occasions, large signs that stated "Alcohol is forbidden" before entering a ceremonial site (M: *ngillatuwe*).

Excessive alcohol consumption is prevalent in the region, and it is common to see men (Mapuche and non-Mapuche) lying drunk in public squares, at bus stops, and on roads. Thus, men consume alcohol in a very visible way. Issues of domestic violence, also prevalent in the region, are associated with alcohol consumption. Alcohol consumption, violence against women within the household, and violence between men in public places were recurring themes of concern among men and women, and among young and old. Along with the above, the stereotype of the Mapuche as lazy and drunk, still present in the press and the national imaginary as has already been discussed, makes the public consumption of alcohol an issue that can generate collective feelings of shame and humiliation, especially among Mapuche men.

Although my contact with the Mapuche Pentecostal world was limited, I met several people who considered themselves "Christians" (they are roughly 30 percent of rural Mapuche).[7] For some of them, this self-designation was not incompatible with participation in Mapuche ritual life. However, for others it was. One of the main reasons they gave as to why they did not participate in Mapuche rituals was the presence of alcohol. Some women, especially middle-aged women, remembered the *ngillatun* ritual as an event in which they experienced fear. Men consumed alcohol uncontrollably. Drunken men used to fight among themselves, sometimes on horseback. Some women I met, and, significantly, their sons and daughters, described it as a relief to have been able to stop participating. Their Church had empowered these women to impose their decision to stop participating in the *ngillatun* ritual. In addition, I met Pentecostals who told me that their Church had saved their fathers from alcohol and changed their fathers completely. Pentecostal movements condemned both alcohol consumption and physical violence against wives. One could argue that the condemnation of alcohol consumption by the Pentecostal movement has generated new negotiating tools for rural Mapuche women (even for those who do not consider themselves "Christians"), as well as a reconfiguration of masculinity among Mapuche rural men. Thus, some men abandon (although not completely) common conducts associated with virility such as alcohol consumption and violence.[8]

In this section, I have explored how ritual action allows for power and moral negotiations to take place within Mapuche society. How, when, and if men should consume alcohol constitutes a terrain for gender and religious negotiations. Ritual action allows for negotiations on which actions are acceptable and which are not within Mapuche ritual life. It also forces people in positions of hierarchical authority, in this case, middle-aged men, to explain their behavior and acknowledge their mistakes in the face of people who are normally under their authority, in this case women and young men and boys.

The *Wetripantü* Ritual and Mapuche Identity at an Individual Level: Becoming a *Longko*

This section aims to account for the individual experience of Mapuche identity in the course of Mapuche ritual life. I have selected the case of Raúl, a middle-aged man who was the *longko* (headman) of a Mapuche community in the Neuquén Province in Argentina. He was a frequent visitor of Machi Carmen, who was acting as the machi of his community. I had met him on several occasions before the *wetripantü* ceremony at the machi's house. To arrive at the machi's house, Raúl had to drive for about seven hours through an Andean border crossing. The journey was long, thus he usually stayed one or two nights at the machi's house (this is a common practice when patients come from far away). Raúl was usually accompanied by his wife and other members of his community, most of them kin.

When I met Raúl and his wife Lucía (about a year before the ritual event described above), they told me that they were coming to see Machi Carmen because they were seeking to recover ritual practices that would bring them closer to a Mapuche identity. They thought they had lost the Mapuche *kimün* (ancestral knowledge) as a consequence of a violent history of war and invasion that had led to the murder of their ancestors. They also thought that the military occupation of the Mapuche territory east of the Andes had been more violent than the war in what is now Chile.[9] They explained that they had not seen a machi born in their community (in fact, in the whole Neuquén province) for more than 120 years. That is why they had to travel to Chile to find a machi. According to them, machi were deliberately targeted and murdered by the Argentinian state's military campaign to gain dominance over Patagonia. Thus, they were left with no machi who could identify and teach young people with the spiritual gift to heal. In the same vein, the *longko* (headmen) had been killed by the invaders so they were left without *longko* who could teach the younger generations. *Longko* Raúl's wife, Lucía, told me the following:

> They [the Argentinian Army] killed the best we had, the machi, the *longko*, all the people who had the *kimün*. Our parents had already lost it [the *kimün*] and they could not communicate it to us. We do not know how to speak the language. All the women's jewelry was stolen by the *wingkas*

> (whites, foreigners). I did not inherit anything from my mum. I'm amazed to see the beautiful jewels of the Chilean Mapuche women. And their beautiful clothes [Mapuche traditional clothing]. I almost feel ashamed we do not know how to dress.
>
> (Araucanía 2017, interview)

During the *wetripantü* ceremony, Raúl did not perform the tasks normally performed by a *longko*. Instead of being next to the *rewe*, leading the ceremony along with the machi, he stayed with people who do not exercise a traditional duty. He did not play any musical instrument, as is common among *longko*, nor did he pray out loud (M: *llellipun*) in Mapudungun. In fact, Raúl did not speak Mapudungun and did not know how to conduct a ritual prayer in the Mapuche language. By then, I knew well that Raúl's legitimacy as a *longko* had been questioned by members of his own community and also by the *longko* of the community of Machi Carmen. Even Machi Carmen herself, who was usually supportive and willing to share her knowledge, became irritated when Raúl did not try to perform as other *longko* did during the *wetripantü* ceremony.

Raúl's incapacity to perform as people expect *longko* to do generated doubts about whether Raúl really came from a *longko* lineage (M: *küpan*). People from the community of Machi Carmen had also found out that Raúl had been elected as *longko* by the people in his community. Being a *longko* is a spiritual gift, thus one must have a *longko* spirit in the family to act legitimately as a *longko*. In this way, being a *longko* is not the same as having a position of political representation (a role that some people call a "political" *longko*). Rather, it is understood as a spiritual duty derived from a spiritual gift. It is not people who choose a *longko* (or a machi), rather a lineage spirit chooses the best person in a family to fulfil a spiritual role. A lineage spirit may skip a generation if it is thought that no one is capable of being an ancestral authority. Thus, the spirit may choose a daughter over a mother, or a son over a father. The succession does not necessarily follow the logic of the firstborn and can be skipped to nephews or nieces instead of sons or daughters. Raúl tried to legitimize his role by claiming that he always knew that his maternal grandfather had been a *longko*. Many Mapuche assume that a *longko* spirit is transmitted mainly through the paternal route (the opposite occurs with machi spirits), so this did not completely dispel the doubts.

Moreover, the machi worried that Raúl did not dream, which generated concern because Raúl, as a *longko*, should receive instructions on how to perform the *ngillatun* ritual and other matters of religious importance through dreams.

Undoubtedly, the most important responsibility of a *longko* today is the realization of the *ngillatun*. *Longko* decide the day on which to conduct the ceremony and oversee ritual activities such as prayers, dancing, and animal sacrifice. During a *ngillatun*, *longko* preside over the ceremony either in the company of other *longko* or a machi. Since I met him, Raúl was worried about events that had taken place during and shortly before and after their last community *ngillatun*. Before the ceremony, many people said the animals were making strange noises at night. Raúl thought that these signs were warning calls indicating that something bad was going to happen during the ceremony, but he did not listen. Raúl explained that, at the ceremony, a bull is traditionally tied to the *rewe* and then it is left in the field until it dies. "That animal must die in the field without anyone touching it," said Raúl. During the ceremony some people saw visions of disfigured animals and became very scared. Also, the bull acted aggressively and, agitated, escaped its tether and gored two people. On top of that, a few days after the ceremony, the animal was found decapitated. This generated great commotion in the community. They only found the head (the rest of the animal's body had disappeared) and decided to bury it in the place where the *ngillatun* ceremony begins, at the *ngillatuwe* or ceremonial site. Raúl was not sure whether that had been the right decision. Moreover, he thought that several misfortunes that had been occurring to his people may have been related to the fact that they were not performing the *ngillatun* correctly.

Machi Carmen said to Raúl that the bull's head must be unearthed while performing a new ceremony. After that, the head must be thrown in a river or some moving water. "What was done to the animal was evil, don't you see?" Machi Carmen told Raúl. Someone meant harm to the community and the bull's head was attached to an evil spirit. Therefore, they needed to get rid of the head, and more importantly, of the evil spirit attached to it. The machi traveled to Argentina and performed the ceremony in which the head of the bull was unearthed. Although that gave Raúl relief for a while, when I saw him at the *wetripantü*, he was anxious and full of doubts about how the next *ngillatun* should be celebrated. Raúl and his community had decided to celebrate a *ngillatun* the following year.

Raúl was also worried about the former *longko*, Felipe, who was still alive, but in a wheelchair. Felipe gave up his role after he got sick and lost the ability to walk. When Felipe renounced his *longko* role, Raúl took over. Raúl and Felipe were not relatives. Raúl told me that his community was no longer interested in *Longko* Felipe. In fact, the last time they celebrated the *ngillatun* ritual people did not go the *longko*'s house, as was common practice. Instead, they headed directly to the *ngillatuwe* (the ceremonial site). Machi Carmen explained to Raúl what he had already suspected: "not to start the ceremony at the *longko*'s house is a big mistake." Then, the machi added that the ceremony should be carried out "as it has always been done, as grandparents did." She also reprimanded Raúl when he recognized that he hardly ever visited Felipe. Raúl should visit Felipe on a regular basis, so he can learn from the old *longko* and gain *kimün*.

Despite constant doubts, there was one element that reinforced Raúl's legitimacy as a *longko*: his eight-year-old son was sick. The child suffered from moments of extreme irritability in which he bit, hit, and shouted incoherent things. Apparently, no environmental factor triggered these episodes. Doctors initially thought it could be a form of epilepsy. However, epilepsy was discarded after performing a comprehensive neurological study. In the Mapuche context, a sickness without medical explanation can be a call (S: *llamado*) from the spirits to people who possess special spiritual gifts. Frequently, these types of sickness (M: *kizu kutran*) appear in childhood. Thus, the unexplained illness of the child could be an indication of the presence of a *longko* spirit in the family, which is trying to turn Raúl's attention to his mistakes as *longko* (and is also calling the child who should grow up to become a *longko* after his father). Raúl's family had previously abandoned the spirit: none of Raúl's maternal uncles exercised their *longko* role. So, the spirit might be very angry.

The Sunday after the *wetripantü*, Raúl and his wife, Lucía, asked the machi to "see the clothes" they had brought that belonged to their son. Machi Carmen, as well as some other machi, can also divine diseases through the inspection of a person's clothes, not only the urine. The machi put the boy's clothes in her *rewe*, together with the urine and clothes of other patients who were still there. In this way, Machi Carmen performed a collective session of divination in which each family (or individual) had their turn. Machi Carmen told Raúl and his wife that they had to perform a prayer (M: *llellipun*) with the child every day to appease the spirit. In addition, Raúl had to learn to exercise his role for the sake of his own family, who were vulnerable to spiritual illnesses and evil spirits. Counter-hexes should be used for protection and Raúl should visit the old *longko*, Felipe, regularly. Thus, Machi Carmen legitimized, in front of several members of Raúl's community, the "real" presence of a *longko* lineage (M: *küpan longko*) in Raúl's family.

Raúl's struggle to become a *longko* is both a struggle to conform to normative ideas about what constitutes a Mapuche *longko* and a struggle to participate in collective processes of creating a Mapuche identity. In this way, he becomes indispensable for the continuity of Mapuche cultural practices, while, at the same time, he experiences radical personal transformations. To be a *longko* implies changes in a person's everyday routine: a *longko* must pray every day, avoid drinking alcohol, avoid being alone. Also, a *longko* is expected to cultivate positive relationships with the spirits of the ancestors so that evil forces can be kept at bay. In addition, a *longko* should treat the elders with respect and learn from them, which explains why Raúl was worried about the lack of interest of his community in the old and sick *longko* who preceded him. Moreover, acts of negligence or irresponsibility can have severe spiritual consequences for a *longko* and his family. Thus, to be a *longko* requires a rigorous and persistent personal commitment, which, in turn, is fundamental for the recreation of a shared Mapuche ritual life and knowledge. In Raúl's case, his commitment is manifested in his constant worries about how to properly perform a *ngillatun* ritual. Also, his commitment is expressed in his constant journeys to visit Machi Carmen and her community to gain *kimün* (ancestral knowledge).

At a personal level, themes already addressed in the previous sections reappear. In this way, to become a *longko* is also a process of creating a Mapuche identity that is a source of personal dignity and self-esteem and, also, a personal contribution to a collective Mapuche identity as a source of shared self-worth.

Conclusions: Ritual Healing and Politics of Identity

Ritual healing transformations are part of larger political and social processes and, thus, are relevant beyond specific illness or medical/spiritual problems. Drawing on Csordas (1999), I have defined three levels of interaction between ritual healing transformations and the politics of Mapuche identity: cultural representations of Mapuche identity, social negotiations between conflicting Mapuche actors, and individual transformations. A Mapuche identity, which is no longer a source of pejorative prejudice but, instead, is invested with pride and self-esteem, is a constant theme throughout all the levels of interaction analyzed. Moreover, the three levels of interaction described are inherently political, in the sense that they portray power struggles to define, delimit, and control what it is to be Mapuche. Thus, ritual healing transformations have a political function and are fundamental to the recovery and preservation of Mapuche ritual life and ways of being, which are threatened by ongoing processes of colonization, expropriation, and marginalization.

At a political level, cultural representations of the *wetripantü* celebrations seek to create cultural difference in a context of rights grounded in state politics of cultural recognition. Mapuche activists try to persuade Chileans that the *wetripantü* celebrations are grounded in scientific and historical knowledge and are, thus, a source of common understanding in Southern American societies. Mapuche identity, then, is raised here as a source of knowledge and adequate understanding that was deliberately attacked by the colonizers. In this way, the theme of a Mapuche identity as a collective source of pride and self-esteem appears here as a struggle to influence and gain recognition from the Chilean state and Chilean society. For instance, Mapuche activists claim that the *wetripantü* ritual should be officially recognized by declaring June 24th as a national holiday.

On a social level, the *wetripantü* celebrations allow for negotiations regarding conflicting Mapuche identities, such as gender and religious identity. At a social level, Mapuche identity does not appear uniform as it did on a political level. Instead, negotiations between conflicting social actors, such as women, men, and Pentecostal Mapuche, problematize Mapuche identity. When, how, and if men should consume alcohol is a vehicle to define, delimit, and control aspects of Mapuche identity, such as masculinity and religiosity. Mapuche men should not consume alcohol while conducting ritual obligations, as alcohol is a foreign introduction deliberately thought to weaken and deprave them. Also, alcohol consumption in the ritual context deprives Mapuche ceremonies of their sacred aspects, transforming them into simply social celebrations to have fun. Therefore, the theme of Mapuche identity as a source of shared dignity and pride is framed here as a preoccupation with how men should behave regarding alcohol consumption in the ritual context and beyond. This occurs in a sociohistorical context in which the image of Mapuche men as alcoholics and violent has been (and continues to be) a frequent way of insulting and belittling the Mapuche.

Lastly, individual participation in the *wetripantü* celebrations links personal experience with a collective Mapuche identity and history. Individuals try to conform to normative ideas about what constitutes being Mapuche. In addition, individuals engage in personal struggles to participate in and influence political processes of community and knowledge making. The theme of a dignified Mapuche identity reappears here as the struggle of a man to become a credible *longko*, responsible for carrying out the *ngillatun* ritual as befits the ritual protocol and as his ancestors did.

Ritual healing efficacy, then, not only refers to an existential function through which aspects of the world and self are thematized so that a person or group can make sense of a problematic situation and explore possible courses of action. Rather, ritual healing efficacy also has a political function, which is manifested through the control over what constitutes a pure or authentic Mapuche identity, which is freed from derogatory prejudice and a source of dignity and self-worth. Self-processes, then, need not be restricted to personal transformations in relation to cultural practices and objects; rather, they can also be understood in relation to collective processes of political identity. Foucault's (e.g., 1980: 55–63) observation that disciplines of power create subjectivities is relevant here. In addition, we also need to explore how individuals can create personal identities that can allow them to participate in and influence collective political processes.

The methodology of defining three different levels of interaction between ritual healing and identity politics makes it impossible to ignore the fact that healing transformations are part of political and historical configurations that transcend the ritual event. Therefore, the possibilities of transformation are constrained (and at the same time made possible) by political conditions that generate power correlations. These power correlations change (or are changed) over time, so ritual transformations must be understood in the context of long-term historical changes and the way individuals are oriented to them. In addition, the proposed methodology allows us to understand ritual healing transformations not only as a resistance to power, which is acted upon individuals (which can lead to the impression that ritual healing is politically futile), but also as inherently political actions that act upon power relationships. Thus, ritual healing actions can be politically productive and generative (acting upon power relationships and not just being acted upon). In the Mapuche case, ritual healing plays a fundamental role in creating Mapuche ways of doing and being that are a source of a personal and collective sense of dignity and self-worth. Thus, state politics of cultural recognition are appropriated and transformed.

In conclusion, ritual healing actions and politics of Mapuche identity interact at three levels: cultural representations of Mapuche identity in Chilean public debates, social negotiations among Mapuche social actors, and individual transformations. These three levels are inherently political in the sense that they constitute power struggles to control what constitutes a proper Mapuche identity. In addition, the idea of a collective Mapuche identity that is the source of self-worth and dignity reappears at all three levels as a structuring cultural theme.

Notes

1. See also Bacigalupo 2016.
2. Alcohol consumption within Indigenous and underprivileged groups has been a widely discussed subject in anthropology. The medicalization of alcoholism has been understood by several authors as directly targeting working classes (and minorities in general) and obscuring the social origins of the problem by blaming individuals and families (e.g., Singer 1986; Waitzkin 1991: 177–90). More recently, researchers have changed the focus from medicalization to biomedicalization, attending to issues of neoliberal citizenship, techno-scientific transformations and commodification. For example, Waldram observed that alcohol has dominated the debates on aboriginal mental health in North America, and that no other topic "has

generated such a combination of perverse curiosity, genuine concern, and outright absurdity, not to mention racism" (2004: 134). Waldram was particularly concerned with the pervasiveness of biological explanations claiming an increased genetic vulnerability to alcohol within Indigenous groups (ibid.: 136), as a way of generalizing and essentializing aboriginal proclivity to alcoholism. In the same vein, Salmon (2010) challenged how Canadian medical authorities have targeted aboriginal women to prevent fetal alcohol spectrum disorder, despite the lack of evidence that the disorder is only due to alcohol and that aboriginal women are at a higher risk of drinking during pregnancy. In Australia, McKnight (2002) tried to explain the "devastating effects" of alcohol on aboriginal communities in the Mornington Islands, as caused by the process of colonization through the loss of cultural practices and aboriginal ways of transmitting social norms and values.

3. Saavedra was trying to reassure authorities in Santiago about the feasibility of the military occupation of Araucanía. As the war progressed, he changed his mind: "A war, initiated by a series of military incursions, will always be destructive, expensive, and—above all else—never ending …" (cited in Crow 2013: 33). Bengoa (1996: 186, my translation) described the war as one of the "darkest pages in Chilean history," one in which "the army entered the territory carrying out a war of extermination, without truce, against the civilian population, women and children, herding animals, burning houses and sown fields … The aim was to provoke terror to force them to capitulate." Crow (2013: 33–34) points out that the brutality of the war was also denounced by local and national newspapers of the time.
4. Villalobos has been excluded from academic debates because his view is racist. Unfortunately, he continues to play a role in public debate. Moreover, during the civic-military dictatorship (1973–1990), Villalobos produced school history textbooks. Thus, although marginal today, his view was dominant very recently. Villalobos' main claim is that there are no Mapuche in contemporary Chile, only *mestizos* who share a Hispanic cultural background.
5. See also Cayuqueo 2011, 2017.
6. People use the term Christian to refer to Pentecostal Christians, and they clearly distinguish them from Catholics and other forms of Christianity. To be a Catholic was not considered necessarily incompatible with a Mapuche religiosity, and most of my friends considered themselves both Catholics and Mapuche. Some people, though, do consider Catholicism as incompatible with a Mapuche religiosity.
7. See Durán (2012) for a recent account of Pentecostalism and the Mapuche in the Araucanía region.
8. Sonia Montecinos (2002) has studied the Pentecostal movement in a poor urban neighborhood in Santiago (La Pintana) from a gender perspective. She describes an emerging masculinity abandoning common signs of virility such as football, alcohol, and violence. At the same time, new femininities emerge that extend their horizons from the household to the religious

community. These changes do not necessarily imply a change in unequal gender relations, but they allow for new possibilities of negotiation.

9. The military occupation of Mapuche territory by the Argentine Republic was called "The Conquest of the Desert" (S: *la Conquista del Desierto*) (1878–1885). Whether or not the Argentinian campaign was more violent is unclear. However, there is a generalized perception among the Mapuche (in Chile and Argentina) today that the Mapuche of Chile are relatively well off both in economic and political terms, in comparison to the Mapuche of Argentina.

Conclusions

This ethnography examined ritual healing efficacy in the Mapuche context from a phenomenological perspective and drew mostly on the work of Thomas Csordas (1990, 1993, 1994a, 1994b). The self was understood as the object of transformation of ritual healing or the locus of efficacy of healing actions. Phenomenologically, the self is a process of constituting a person and their world with specific attributes and characteristics according to themes, constraints, and values of the broader social context. These processes of self-objectification are open-ended, indeterminate, and relational and they occur every time the self engages in a relational situation. Nevertheless, self-processes occur within cultural and historical constraints, which explain both the sense of continuity of the self and limits of possible transformations. Self-processes depend on the human capacity of reflexivity through which they end in reflexive conceptualizations. However, they start in pre-reflexive bodily transformations, which are experienced as immediate and spontaneous.

Here, I focused on techniques that deliberately attempt to produce changes that are experienced as immediate and spontaneous, or not mediated by deliberative and effortful cognitive processes. In this manner, I explored ethnographically the way in which ritual healing techniques orient the body toward specific themes and situations, so self-process can move from indeterminacy to orientation and objectification. Special importance was given to the way in which Mapuche shamans or machi use ritual techniques that direct attention toward specific themes or situations; induce affective states, usually negative, such as fear and sadness; alert the senses through different bodily techniques, such as singing, massaging, and dancing; and promote the active involvement of the patient or the community in the search for both the cause and the cure of illness and misfortune. In this way, this work explored how machi transform somatic and affective experience through the utilization of various ritual techniques. In addition, the techniques machi use are embedded in cultural practices of healing, which direct transformations according to specific cultural themes and meaning.

The understanding of the self as a never-ending process of becoming a self is relevant to the question about medical efficacy. These processes carry with them potentialities of experiential transformations. Also, therapeutic techniques can alter, divert and redirect processes of self- transformations according to specific values and beliefs. To posit efficacy on shifts of orientation in processes of self-objectification gives therapeutic techniques great possibilities of producing effective changes. Moreover, efficacy, in this way understood, relies on the performative structure of the ritual act of healing and not only on systems of symbols superimposed into the therapeutic action. Transformation can then be understood as occurring as a direct result of ritual healing action (Hsu 2015; Kapferer 2004). This is not to say that ritual healing action is not constrained by cultural meaning that transcends the social interaction within the therapeutic encounter. But, within specific social constraints, therapeutic action between social actors has an internal capacity for transformation.

A fundamental preoccupation of my interlocutors was the fact that some machi can really know illness and misfortune and their treatment, while others may just be pretending. My interlocutors framed this concern by saying that some machi are real and some machi are fake. Knowing who is (and who is not) a real machi was a constant source of concern for the people I worked with. On a doctrinal level, a real machi is a person with the spiritual gift to heal through knowledge received from a *pülli* (lineage spirit). Machi knowledge (or machi *kimun*) is received directly from the spiritual world through different signs, such as intuitions, *perimontun* (visions), *peuma* (dreams), and *küymin* (ritual trance). A machi must learn how to interpret the spirit's messages so they can become a guide for healing action.

On a practical level, the question of who is a real machi is a complex one and it deals with multiple issues, such as the moral disposition of a healer (whether a healer uses their powers to harm or for their own personal gain), power and wealth, personality and charisma, and also the authenticity of tradition and its validation in the eyes of the state. However, I mostly focused on aspects of this

Mapuche preoccupation that are related to the use of transformative techniques that can effectively see or know illness, make evil spirits visible so they can be neutralized, and make "spirits from the past" present, so they can deliver a message to the community. Therefore, a real machi is one who can see illness through different divinatory techniques, make evil spirits visible, so they can be identified, neutralized and disposed of, and act as a medium of the spiritual world.

As I have shown, there were two fundamental characteristics that my interlocutors thought made a machi a real machi. First, a real machi has the spiritual ability to see illness and misfortune through different divinatory techniques, most commonly through the visual inspection of a patient's bottled urine or *willentun*. In the Mapuche context, seeing is related to knowing and understanding. Thus, when people said "a machi must see the urine" or "I need a machi to see my urine," they were expressing the expectation that a machi can know both what their problem is and what the possible solution to it is. Secondly, machi preside over community ceremonies, such as the *ngillatun* ritual, which aim to maintain the wellbeing of the group through direct communication with the spiritual world. Machi are the only individuals who can experience *küymin* or trance, or the ritually induced possession of a machi by the spirit of a deceased shaman. Through *küymin*, "spirits from the past" can be made present and deliver a message to an individual, family, or community. Machi, then, are the depositaries of *kimün* (ancestral knowledge) regarding Mapuche ritual life and spirituality and Mapuche ways of dealing with illness, misfortune, and hardship. Therefore, machi practices are key in the recreation, preservation, and endless transmission of the Mapuche world.

As stated above, machi can see illnesses through *pewtun* techniques, which most commonly occur in the form of the visual inspection of a patient's bottled urine (*willentun*). *Pewtun* divinatory techniques consist of the utilization of an open-ended, tentative, and apparently aimless speech on the part of the machi. The machi speech does not seek to generate a coherent system of meaning, rather it promotes an active patient, willing to creatively engage with an existential situation. In this way, the machi's words, together with their gestures, pauses, and sharp looks, increase tension and focus attention, guiding the patient toward the exploration of possible causes of suffering.

Symptoms, such as headache or impaired vision; conditions of the body, such as the weakening of the bones or the swelling of internal organs; together with emotions, such as sadness; or life experiences, such as excessive work, are enumerated. Machi's enumerations of alternative explanations to a problem seem to be building up uncertainty and possibilities, rather than giving one definite answer. Thus, the patient must be an active participant in the process of seeking an explanation for their problems. The patient contributes through gestures and words of approval and disapproval, guiding the machi to which topics to abandon and which topics to pursue. In addition, the patient can contribute to the search for an explanation through an intense emotional response to the description of negative emotions such as sadness, or adverse experiences such as not feeling loved or valued.

Pewtun techniques also involve the induction of affective dispositions, which are usually negative, such as fear and sadness. Affective dispositions are induced by increasing the tension and expectation of what a machi might see and say. Patients commonly fear they might be the victims of witchcraft or that someone might have harmed them (S: *me hicieron un daño*), because this is something machi usually divine. Machi increase tension and fear with sharp looks at the patient's urine, while shaking it or slowly moving it, and long silences. In addition, some machi use pre-constructed narratives on emotional suffering, which can elicit an emotional response on the part of the patient. These narratives are gendered and give meaning to emotional suffering. Some machi use narratives based on sadness due to not being valued or loved in the case of women, and narratives about feelings of humiliation and hard work in the case of men. Intense negative affective responses can produce a moment of synchronicity (Hsu 2005), in which all the participants focus attention into one emotional response or painful experiential situation. The technical creation of synchronicity alerts the senses, the emotions, and the attention, promoting active participation in the elaboration of explanations and solutions. Also, synchronicity can generate an experience of connectedness through the generation of shared experiential situations.

Once the patient is actively engaged with the healing situation, machi and patient are usually able to reflexively construct a dialogue and give meaning to a painful situation. Through this dialogue between machi and patient (and sometimes the patient's family) both the cause of and the solution to an affliction are negotiated and discussed. The dialogue between machi and patient, although it usually leads to some definitive understanding of a problematic situation and possible courses of action, remains ambiguous and open-ended. In this way, problems detected may change in subsequent consultations or even during one single consultation, and there is usually more than one single topic discussed during one *pewtun* divination. In addition, machi usually advise the patient to come back to make sure the treatment is having a positive effect. Thus, treatments are prolonged in time, and the cause of affliction is a constant source of new explorations and negotiations.

Some of the healing actions described above produce changes in bodily and affective experience that are not mediated by reconfigurations of symbolic meaning. These bodily and affective changes occur independently of conscious cognitive processes and are, thus, experienced as sudden and involuntary. Bodily transformations during a *pewtun* session may be therapeutic in at least two ways, which are inter-related. First, they enhance the experience of trans-individual connection through the creation of shared somatic and affective experience. Second, since they promote awareness and volition, they predispose a person to new dispositions to everyday experience (Csordas 1993; Desjarlais 1996; Devisch 1990; Hsu 2005, 2015; Seremetakis 1998). Moreover, healing bodily transformations provide the experiential ground from which the reflexive understanding of a situation is elaborated. Therefore, only after the patient is actively engaged, through embodied and spontaneous bodily transformations, can machi and patient create a common understanding and agree on possible courses of action.

In this way, *pewtun* sessions can be understood as being targeted at self-processes (Csordas 1994a). Stated differently, self-processes can be understood as the object of transformation of *pewtun* techniques. Self-processes start in bodily pre-reflexive experience, which is sudden and involuntary, and end in self-objectification, or the reflexive understanding of a problematic situation or one's adverse circumstances and possible solutions. Reflexive understanding, then, is grounded in the body and its practices, habits, and skills. Also, the reflexive understanding of a situation comes to be in the fitting together of somatic and emotional experience, cultural objects of the milieu, and cultural practices structured by the habitus (Csordas 1990).

In the case of the *pewtun* ritual, somatic and affective experience usually happens in the form of focusing attention on the bottled urine and the machi speech, increasing feelings of expectations regarding what the machi may say and emotional responses to the machi's words. Relevant cultural objects of the milieu are common ways in which people understand illness and suffering. In the Mapuche context, the agents of affliction are usually evil spirits. Also, the agents of afflictions may be spirits from the past, who are trying to warn people regarding the consequences of spiritual transgressions. Spiritual afflictions are also related to human moral transgressions, such as not engaging with Mapuche ritual life or Mapuche norms of relating to nature, such as cultivating the land on a ceremonial site, cutting down native trees, not teaching the children to speak the Mapuche language, and either not participating or participating irresponsibly in Mapuche ceremonies. Furthermore, illness can derive from unloving relationships and from experiences of humiliation and discrimination of people who are in the margins of society. Somatic and affective transformations are elaborated according to the cultural themes described above through *pewtun* techniques. In turn, *pewtun* techniques are structured through the Mapuche habitus, which can explain why certain somatic experiences have immediate meaning, without the necessity of further explanation, or why certain narratives on emotional pain can promote a rapid and intense emotional response.

Machi are the only type of practitioners who can effectively deal with evil spirits or *wekufe*. For some of my Mapuche interlocutors, this was the most important reason why machi should continue to exist. In addition, evil spirits are usually the most common cause that mobilizes non-Mapuche people to seek the help of a machi. Dealing with evil spirits is a marginal activity that usually puts a machi's reputation at risk. Because machi deal with evil forces, they are usually suspected of being *kalku* (witches) themselves or using tricks and being dishonest for their own economic gain. Therefore, the capacity to deal with evil forces is both a source of power, wealth, and prestige, and a source of marginality and suspicion. Machi need to navigate this complex paradox. However, when they can deal with evil spirits effectively, they can use the wealth and power gained to increase their reputation and social legitimacy. For instance, machi can use their money to organize traditional Mapuche ceremonies, in which they are the mediums of benevolent spirits from the past. These ceremonies are morally positive, instead of the more morally ambiguous ritual action directed at evil forces. Thus, machi can use their own marginality as a source of power, control, and money.

When evil spirits are the suspected agents of affliction, a machi needs to make them visible to prove they are, indeed, the cause of suffering and also to direct proper healing action against them. Making evil spirits visible is achieved through self-processes in which sensory and affective experience becomes the "materialization," as my interlocutors used to say, of evil forces. Self-processes occur through forms of imaginative seeing such as visual, auditory, and haptic images, and negative emotions, such as fear. Here, somatic and affective experience, evil spirits as objects of the Mapuche milieu, and the Mapuche habitus come together to create the meaningful experience of the collective seeing of evil forces, so they can later be contained and disposed of. Stated otherwise, the imaginative communal seeing of evil spirits is a mode of self-processes through which the cause of an affliction is objectified, and proper healing action can then be taken against it.

Imagination is fundamental in Mapuche ritual healing and machi promote it in different sensorial forms, such as visual images, auditory images, and emotional experience. Here, imagination is something that the body does, an act, in the form of sensorial and affective experience. In this way, imagination is close to perception, although it supposes the experience of something as possible rather than actual (Jansen 2010; Sartre 2004). Machi inculcate imagination through different techniques to promote shifts in orientation of the body toward specific objects, themes, and values. This is achieved through the imaginative seeing of an illness and a problem in a patient's bottled urine or through the communal seeing of evil spirits, as I have shown.

Every time a machi engages with ritual action, they are facing the question of whether they are real or not. Do they really have the knowledge to understand and treat illness and misfortune? Are they really a good healer? The answer to the question of who is a real machi is usually not a definitive one, rather machi constantly face the possibility of failure and doubts regarding their healing powers.

Also, they can restore trust in their powers despite partial failure and doubts. A machi´s performance may generate doubts regarding the healer's powers if they fail to carry out actions according to the ritual conventions, thus revealing a lack of *kimün* (ancestral knowledge). A machi can also be judged negatively if serious mishaps and unexpected events occur during ritual action. In this way, ritual failure can be understood as a performance failure (Grimes 1990; Schieffelin 1996, 2007), in which the authenticity of the performer is what is at stake (and not the ritual itself). A machi's performance may be imperfect due to several reasons, such as crying while in trance and, thus, generating doubts regarding the presence of the machi spirit. Because spirits do not cry in the way humans do, the crying of a machi while in trance questions the authenticity of the machi as a medium of their spirit. The importance of carrying out ritual actions as befits the ritual conventions is related to the need to "recover" and protect Mapuche knowledge and spirituality, which is threatened by ongoing processes of colonization. In this manner, machi are expected to be the depositaries of ancestral tradition and wisdom, and their failure to do so threatens the continuity of Mapuche ritual life and spirituality.

Machi can also fail if they cannot interpret the messages they receive from the spirits. Spiritual signs should guide healing action and inform a machi's practice. However, machi should learn to understand the messages from the sprits. Machi initiates, then, engage in a learning process about how to interpret spiritual signs and transform them into directions for effectively engaging in ritual action. The ethnographic observations presented here show that a machi who can successfully perform makes the spirits present through ritual action, rather than just being the passive receiver of a spiritual message. In this manner, if a *machil* or machi initiate passively waits for a clear spiritual message to come, they end up feeling as if they lack inspiration and are incapable of performing as a machi. The spirits cannot be present before a machi's actions, because they are invisible. Thus, they can only become visible or present through the skillful actions of a real machi. To make the spirits present, a machi needs to "simulate" (Kendall 1996: 50) the spirits, talk for them, sing for them, and perform for them. If, instead, a machi initiate waits for the spirits to come before performing, Mapuche ritual healing cannot be initiated. Therefore, inspiration, in the Mapuche context, refers to the capacity of making the spirits present or making the agents of affliction visible through healing action.

Machi are not only healers, rather they also exercise a role as community builders and transmitters of tradition and cultural practices. Besides presiding over ritual healing events, machi also preside over traditional ceremonies that aim to preserve Mapuche ritual life and Mapuche ways of relating and maintaining balance with the spiritual world. In these ceremonies, particularly in the *ngillatun* ritual, machi experience *küymin* or ritual trance. Through *küymin*, a group of people can receive a direct message from "spirits from the past." The spirits usually provide moral guidance regarding what constitutes proper behavior in the Mapuche context and what constitutes proper ways of relating with other people, nature, and the spiritual world. The spirits also provide explanations regarding the cause of illness and misfortune, together with possible courses of action to prevent and treat them. Moreover, the spirits constitute an enactment of the past in the present, which is fundamental in Mapuche ways of creating a shared memory or a common history. In this way, machi are fundamental to the transmission of cultural practices and the creation of shared feelings of belonging to a community.

Mapuche medical practices, then, can be understood as part of larger struggles for the maintenance, recovery, and permanent recreation of a shared Mapuche identity and memory. Machi are the depositaries of *kimün* (ancestral knowledge) because they can directly communicate with the spirits of the ancestors through dreams, visions, and *küymin* (ritual trance). Thus, machi are a vehicle for the enactment and transmission of Mapuche past and memory and its permanent re-creation in the present. In this manner, machi presiding over traditional ceremonies and transmitting messages from the spiritual world to the community is fundamental to maintaining Mapuche ritual life and the communities that make it possible. Machi practices, then, can be understood as a political resistance to colonization and marginalization and as a way of recovering self-esteem, dignit,y and self-worth, as many of my Mapuche friends explicitly stated.

Then, ritual healing interacts with politics of Mapuche identity. These interactions occur at a political, social, and individual level. The exploration of interactions at different levels allows us to methodologically disentangle the relations between the personal and the collective, and the macropolitical and the micropolitical. At a political level, or at the level of representational practices, Mapuche discourses on ritual healing create a Mapuche identity that is differentiated from the rest of Chilean society. Cultural difference is a source of state recognition and cultural rights, and also of shared feelings of pride and self-esteem. On a social level, ritual action offers a way of negotiating conflicting identities, roles, and expectations within Mapuche society. Thus, ritual action offers possibilities for dealing with social conflict and hierarchies in constructive ways. On an individual level, engaging in ritual healing actions allows for the creation of a personal identity in relation to a shared Mapuche identity and memory. For some individuals, an illness episode is interpreted as a spiritual call to become a Mapuche ancestral authority, such as a machi or a *longko* (headman). When this is the case, individuals can experience radical personal transformations and a sense of becoming a new self.

Machi medical practices are embedded in broader political Mapuche struggles for knowledge, authenticity, and tradition. In this way, ritual healing practices are part of political strategies of enhancing cultural difference in the context of state politics of cultural recognition and rights. At the same time, Mapuche politics also claim to understand Mapuche ways of being in Mapuche terms (and not only in the terms the state is willing to recognize and accept as valid). For example, Mapuche activists claim they can know the past through the trance of a machi or the dreams of Mapuche people. In this way, they can claim the precolonial origin of their collective ritual ceremonies. In addition, illnesses and death usually derive from human transgressions in the way people relate to the natural environment and the spiritual beings it contains. Mapuche claim they should engage in Mapuche ways of relating to nature through their own knowledge of nature and their own knowledge of the ways in which the natural world relates to the social and the spiritual worlds. In this manner, Mapuche ritual action can both reconstruct Mapuche memory and re-establish balance between the social, the natural, and the spiritual world.

In conclusion, a real machi is one who can see or know illness and misfortune and make them visible to the sufferer. Seeing is achieved through shifts in orientation in self-processes. These shifts occur through the technical manipulation of the senses, the induction of affective states, and the promotion of attentiveness and awareness regarding an existential situation. Once the problem or the agents of affliction have been made visible, people can construct meaning around them and discuss possible courses of action. In this way, the understanding of the cause of an affliction and possible solutions is grounded in bodily transformations that are experienced as immediate and spontaneous and are not mediated by conscious cognitive processes. However, bodily transformations are of tremendous significance for the creation of reflexive meaning in an experiential way. In addition, a real machi is one who can make spirits from the past present through *küymin* or ritual trance. To achieve this goal, machi must perform for the spirits. Stated differently, machi must act for the spirits, usually in the form of a sung prayer and other actions, which can then become a source of inspiration and knowledge. Because machi are a direct vehicle for communicating with spirits from the past, they are fundamental to Mapuche political struggles for identity and memory.

References

Amestica, J., and C. Aldunate. 2013. "Carmen Aldunate: 'Los Mapuches Son Violentos Porque Es Más Entretenido y Fácil'." *The Clinic*, [online]. Retrieved 14 June 2019 from www.theclinic.cl/2013/01/12/carmen-aldunate-los-mapuches-son-violentos-porque-es.

Asad, T. 1997. "Remarks on the Anthropology of the Body." In *Religion and the Body*, ed. S. Coakley, 42–52. Cambridge: Cambridge University Press.

Bacigalupo, A.M. 2001. *La Voz del Kultrun en la Modernidad: Tradición y Cambio en la Terapéutica de Siete Machi Mapuche*. Santiago: Ediciones Universidad de Chile.

Bacigalupo, A.M. 2007. *Shamans of the Foye Tree*. Austin: University of Texas Press.

Bacigalupo, A.M. 2016. *Thunder Shaman: Making History with Mapuche Spirits in Chile and Patagonia*. Austin: University of Texas Press.

Baquedano, M. 2004. *La Batalla de Ralco*. Santiago: Instituto de Ecología Política, Lom Ediciones.

Bartlett, J. 2018. "Chile: Four Police Officers Arrested Over Fatal Shooting of Indigenous Man." *The Guardian*, [online]. Retrieved 26 November 2019. www.theguardian.com/world/2018/nov/29/chile.

Basadre, P. 2018. "Muerte de Catrillanca: CIPER Revela en Exclusiva Tres de los Videos que Grabó Carabineros." CIPER, [online]. Retrieved 26 November 2019. https://ciperchile.cl/2018/12/19/muerte-de.

Bengoa, J. 1996. *Historia del Pueblo Mapuche*. 3rd ed. Santiago: Ediciones Sur.

Bengoa, J. 2002. *Historia de un Conflicto: El Estado y los Mapuches en el Siglo XX*. Santiago: Editorial Planeta.

Bengoa, J. 2012. "Memoria y Rito: El Ngillatun y el We Tripantü entre los Mapuche." In *Mapuche: Procesos, Políticas y Culturas en el Chile del Bicentenario*, ed. J. Bengoa. Santiago: Catalonia.

Bengoa, J., and N. Caniguan. (2012). "Los Mapuche y el Bicentenario." In *Mapuche: Procesos, Políticas y Culturas en el Chile del Bicentenario*, ed. J. Bengoa. Santiago: Catalonia.

Berger, H. 1987. "Bodies and Texts." *Representations*, 13(17): 144–6.

Bourdieu, P. 1977. *Outline of a Theory of Practice*. Cambridge: Cambridge University Press.

Bourdieu, P. 1986. *Distinction: A Social Critique of the Judgement of Taste*. London: Routledge.

Briones, C. 2003. "Re-membering the Dis-membered: A Drama About Mapuche and Anthropological Cultural Production in Three Scenes." *Journal of Latin American Anthropology*, 8(3): 31–58.

Cayuqueo, P. 2011. "We Tripantü." *The Clinic*, [online]. Retrieved 9 January 2020 from www.theclinic.cl/2011/06/27/we-tripantu/.

Cayuqueo, P. 2017. *Historia Secreta Mapuche*. Santiago: Catalonia.

Collier, G. 1994. "The New Politics of Exclusion: Antecedents to the Rebellion in Mexico." *Dialectical Anthropology*, 19(1): 1–44.

Collins, R. 2004. *Interaction Ritual Chains*. Princeton: Princeton University Press.

Cooper, J. 1946. "The Araucanians." In *Handbook of South American Indians*, ed. J. Steward, 687–760. Washington: Smithsonian Institution.

Course, M. 2011. *Becoming Mapuche: Person and Ritual in Indigenous Chile*. Urbana: University of Illinois Press.

Crossley, N. 1996. "Body-Subject/Body-Power: Agency, Power and Inscription in Foucault and Merleau-Ponty." *Body & Society*, 2(1): 99–116.

Crow, J. 2013. *The Mapuche in Modern Chile: A Cultural History*. Gainesville: University Press of Florida.

Crow, J. 2014. "From Araucanian Warriors to Mapuche Terrorists: Contesting Discourses of Gender, Race, and Nation in Modern Chile (1810–2010)." *Journal of Iberian and Latin American Studies*, 20(1): 75–101.

Csordas, T. 1990. "Embodiment as a Paradigm for Anthropology." *Ethos*, 18(1): 5–47.

Csordas, T. 1993. "Somatic Modes of Attention." *Cultural Anthropology*, 8(2): 135–56.

Csordas, T. 1994a. *The Sacred Self: A Cultural Phenomenology of Charismatic Healing*. Berkeley: University of California Press.

Csordas, T. 1994b. "Introduction." In *Embodiment and Experience*, ed. T. Csordas, 1–24. Cambridge: Cambridge University Press.

Csordas, T. 1999. "Ritual Healing and the Politics of Identity in Contemporary Navajo Society." *American Ethnologist*, 26(1): 3–23.

Cuyul, A. 2013. "La Política de Salud Chilena y el Pueblo Mapuche. Entre el Multiculturalismo y la Autonomía Mapuche en Salud." *Salud Problema*, [online] 14: 21–33. Retrieved 23 February 2020 from https://uam-xochimilco.academia.edu/AndresCuyul.

Cuyul, A. 2015. "Pensar la Autonomía Mapuche en Salud, o la Persistencia del Dispositivo Intercultural." Mapuexpress, [online]. Retrieved 4 December 2019 from www.mapuche.info/?kat=11&sida=5842.

Degarrod, L.N. 1998. "Female Shamanism and the Mapuche Transformation into Christian Chilean Farmers." *Religion*, 28(4): 339–50.

De la Cadena, M. 2010. "Indigenous Cosmopolitics in the Andes: Conceptual Reflections Beyond Politics." *Cultural Anthropology*, 25(2): 34–370.

De la Cadena, M. 2015. *Earth Beings: Ecologies of Practice Across Andean Worlds*. Durham: Duke University Press.

Desjarlais, R. 1996. "Presence." In *The Performance of Healing*, ed. C. Laderman and M. Roseman, 143–65. London: Routledge.

Devisch R. 1990. "The Human Body as Vehicle for Emotions Among the Yaka of Zaire." In *Personhood and Agency: The Experience of Self and Other in African Cultures*, ed. M. Jackson and I. Karp, 115–33. Uppsala: Uppsala University.

Douglas, M. 1966. *Purity and Danger: An Analysis of Concepts of Pollution and Taboo*. London: Routledge and Kegan Paul.

Douglas, M. 1970. *Natural Symbols: Explorations in Cosmology*. London: Barrie and Rockliffe.

Durán, D. 2012. "Pentecostalismo Mapuche." In *Mapuche: Procesos, Políticas y Culturas en el Chile del Bicentenario*, ed. J. Bengoa, Santiago: Catalonia.

Evans-Pritchard, E.E. 1976[1937]. *Witchcraft, Oracles and Magic Among the Azande*. Oxford: Clarendon Press.

Faron, L. 1997[1964]. *Antüpaiñamko: Moral y ritual mapuche. Traducido del inglés por P. Mege*. Santiago: Ediciones Mundo.

Favret-Saada, J. 1980. *Deadly Words: Witchcraft in the Bocage*. Cambridge: Cambridge University Press.

Foerster, R., and S. Montecinos. 1988. *Organizaciones, Líderes y Contiendas Mapuches (1900–1970)*. Santiago: Ediciones CEM.

Foucault, M. 1980. "Body-Power." In *Power/Knowledge: Selected Interviews and Other Writings 1972–1977*, ed. C. Gordon, 55–63. Brighton: Harvester.

Frank, J. 1963. *Persuasion and Healing: A Comparative Study of Psychotherapy*. New York: Schocken Books.

Gabriel, J. 1994. "Initiating a Movement: Indigenous, Black and Grassroots Struggles in the Americas." *Race and Class*, 35(3): 1–17.

Geissler, P., and R. Prince. 2010. "Persons, Plants and Relations: Treating Childhood Illness in a Western Kenyan Village." In *Plants, Health and Healing: On the Interface of Ethnobotany and Medical Anthropology*, ed. E. Hsu and H. Stephen, 179–223. New York: Berghahn Books.

Good, B.J. 1994. *Medicine, Rationality and Experience*. Cambridge: Cambridge University Press.

Good, B.J., and M.J. DelVecchio-Good. 1993. "Learning Medicine: The Constructing of Medical Knowledge at Harvard Medical School." In *Knowledge, Power, and Practice: The Anthropology of Medicine and Everyday Life*, ed. S. Lindenbaum and M. Lock, 81–107. Cambridge: Cambridge University Press.

Grimes, R. 1990. *Ritual Criticism: Case Studies in its Practice, Essays on its Theory*. Columbia: University of South Carolina Press.

Hale, C. 1994. "Between Che Guevara and the Pachamama: Mestizos, Indians and Identity Politics in the Anti-Quincentenary Campaign." *Critique of Anthropology*, 14(1): 9–39.

Hale, C. 1997. "Cultural Politics of Identity." *Annual Review of Anthropology*, 261(1): 567–90.

Hale, C. 2005. "Neoliberal Multiculturalism: The Remaking of Cultural Rights and Racial Dominance in Central America." *Political and Legal Anthropology Review*, 28(1): 10–28.

Haraway, D. 1991. *Simians, Cyborgs and Women: The Reinvention of Nature*. New York: Routledge.

Hobsbawm, E.J., and T.O. Ranger. 1983. *The Invention of Tradition*. Cambridge: Cambridge University Press.

Hsu, E. 2005. "Acute Pain Infliction as Therapy." *Etnofoor*, 18(1): 78–96.

Hsu, E. 2008. "The Senses and the Social: An Introduction." *Ethnos*, 73(4): 433–43.

Hsu, E. 2010. *Pulse Diagnosis in Early Chinese Medicine: The Telling Touch*. Cambridge: Cambridge University Press.

Hsu, E. 2015. "Sensory Experience in Therapeutics. Series of lectures. Option Course on Medical Anthropology." University of Oxford, Hilary Term.

Humphrey, C., and J. Laidlaw. 1994. *The Archetypal Actions of Ritual: A Theory of Ritual Illustrated by the Jain Rite of Worship*. Oxford: Clarendon Press.

Hüsken, U. 2007. *When Rituals Go Wrong: Mistakes, Failure and the Dynamics of Ritual*. Leiden: Brill.

Ingold, T. 2000. *The Perception of the Environment: Essays on Livelihood, Dwelling and Skill*. London, New York: Routledge.

Instituto Nacional de Estadísticas (INE). 2025. "Síntesis de Resultados Censo 2024. INE." Retrieved 11 October 2025 from https://censo2024.ine.gob.cl/resultados/.

International Labour Organization (ILO). 1989. "C169-Indigenous and Tribal Peoples Convention." *ILO*, [online]. Retrieved 2 April 2020 from www.ilo.org/dyn/normlex/en/f?p=NORMLEXPUB:12100:0::NO::P12100_ILO_CODE: C169.

Itzhak, N. 2015. "Making Selves and Meeting Others in Neo-Shamanic Healing." *Ethos*, 43(3): 286–310.

Jackson, M. 2012. *Lifeworlds: Essays in Existential Anthropology*. Chicago, London: University of Chicago Press.

Jansen, J. 2010. "Phenomenology, Imagination and Interdisciplinary Research." In *Handbook of Phenomenology and Cognitive Science*, ed. D. Schmicking and S. Gallagher, 141–58. Dordrecht: Springer.

Jansen, J. 2018. "Imagination De-Naturalized: Phantasy, the Imaginary, and Imaginative Ontology." In *The Oxford Handbook of the History of Phenomenology*, ed. D. Zahavi, 676–95. Oxford: Oxford University Press.

Kapferer, B. 1991. *A Celebration of Demons: Exorcism and the Aesthetics of Healing in Sri Lanka*. Washington: Smithsonian Institution Press.

Kapferer, B. 2004. "Ritual Dynamics and Virtual Practice: Beyond Representation and Meaning." *Social Analysis*, 48(2): 35–54.

Kendall, L. 1996. "Initiating Performance: The Story of Chini, a Korean Shaman." In *The Performance of Healing*, ed. C. Laderman and M. Roseman, 17–58. London: Routledge.

Kirmayer, L. 1992. The Body's Insistence on Meaning: Metaphor as Presentation and Representation in Illness Experience." *Medical Anthropology Quarterly New Series*, 6(4): 323–46.

Kleinman, A. 1973. "Medicine's Symbolic Reality: On a Central Problem in the Philosophy of Medicine." *Inquiry*, 16(1–4): 206–13.

Kleinman, A. 1980. *Patients and Healers in the Context of Culture: An Exploration of the Borderland between Anthropology, Medicine, and Psychiatry*. Berkeley, London: University of California Press.

Kleinman, A. 1988. *The Illness Narratives: Suffering, Healing and the Human Condition*. New York: Basic Books.

Kohn, E. 2007. "How Dogs Dream: Amazonian Natures and the Politics of Transspecies Engagement." *American Ethnologist*, 34(1): 3–24.

Kohn, E. 2013. *How Forests Think: Toward an Anthropology Beyond the Human*. Berkeley: University of California Press.

Kristensen, D. 2019. *Patients, Doctors and Healers: Medical Worlds Among the Mapuche in Southern Chile*. Cham, Switzerland: Palgrave Macmillan.

Lenz, R. 1896. *Introducción a los Estudios Araucanos: Apéndice Bibliográfico*. Santiago: Imprenta Cervantes.

Lévi-Strauss, C. 1963. *Structural Anthropology*. New York: Basic Books.

Lewis, G. 1980. *Day of Shining Red: An Essay on Understanding Ritual*. Cambridge: Cambridge University Press.

Lewis, G. 2000. *A Failure of Treatment*. Oxford: Oxford University Press.

Lewis, I.M. 2003. *Ecstatic Religion: A Study of Shamanism and Spirit Possession*. London, New York: Routledge.

Lindquist, G. 2005. "Bringing the Soul Back to the Self: Soul Retrieval in Neo-shamanism." In *Ritual in its Own Right: Exploring the Dynamics of Transformation*, ed. D. Handelman and G. Lindquist, 157–73. New York, Oxford: Berghahn Books.

Mallon, F. 2005. *Courage Tastes of Blood: The Mapuche Community of Nicolás Aillío and the Chilean State, 1906–2001*. Durham: Duke University Press.

Marileo, A. 2008. "¿We-Tripantü o Año Nuevo en el Hemisferio Sur?" *Mapuche Foundation FOLIL*, [online]. Retrieved 9 January 2020 from www.mapuche.nl/espanol/wetripantu0806.html.

Marimán, P., S. Caniuqueo, J. Millalén, and R. Levil. (2006) *¡... Escucha, Winka ...! Cuatro Ensayos de Historia Nacional Mapuche y Un Epílogo sobre el Futuro*. Santiago: LOM Ediciones.

McKnight D. 2002. *From Drinking to Hunting: The Devastating Effects of Alcohol on an Australian Aboriginal Community*. London: Routledge.

Merleau-Ponty, M. 2012[1945]. *The Phenomenology of Perception*. London: Routledge. 226.

Merz, B. 2007. "When a Goddess Weeps—Ritual Failure or Failed Performance? A Case Study from Nepal." In *When Rituals Go Wrong: Mistakes, Failures and the Dynamics of Ritual*, ed. U. Hüsken, 209–22. Leiden: Brill.

Michelson, C., and P. Cayuqueo. 2017. "Pedro Cayuqueo: 'No Éramos una Tribu que Andaba a Poto Pelao, Comiendo Moras'." *The Clinic*, [online]. Retrieved 9 January 2020 from www.theclinic.cl/2017/10/17/pedro-cayuqueo-no-eramos-una-tribu-andabamos-potopelado-comiendo-moras/.

Moerman, D. 2002. *Meaning, Medicine and the "Placebo Effect."* Cambridge: Cambridge University Press.

Montecinos, S. 2002. "Nuevas Feminidades y Masculinidades: Una Mirada de Género al Mundo Evangélico de La Pintana." *Estudios Públicos*, [online] Volume 87: 73–103. Retrieved 31 March 2020 from www.cepchile.cl/cep/estudios-publicos/n-61-a-la-90/estudios-publicos-n-87/nuevasfeminidades-y-masculinidades-una-mirada-de-genero-al-mundo.

Núñez de Pineda y Bascuñán, F. 1863[1673]. *Cautiverio Feliz y Razón de las Guerras Dilatadas de Chile*. Santiago: Imprenta el Ferrocarril.

Ots, T. 1994. "The Silenced Body—the Expressive Leib: On the Dialectic of Mind and Life in Chinese Cathartic Healing." In *Embodiment and Experience*, ed. T. Csordas, 116–38. Cambridge: Cambridge University Press.

Ozawa-de Silva, C. 2006. *Psychotherapy and Religion in Japan: The Japanese Introspection Practice of Naikan*. London: Routledge.

Pandolfi, M. 2007. "Memory Within the Body: Women's Narrative and Identity in a Southern Italian Village." In *Beyond the Body Proper: Reading the Anthropology of Material Life*, ed. M. Lock and J. Farquhar, 451–8. Durham, London: Duke University Press.

Parkin, D. 1985. "Introduction." In *The Anthropology of Evil*, ed. D. Parkin, 1–25. Oxford: Blackwell.

Parkin, D. 1991. "Simultaneity and Sequencing in the Oracular Speech of Kenyan Diviners." In *African Divination Systems: Ways of Knowing*, ed. P. Peek, 173–89. Bloomington: Indiana University Press.

Pinto, J. 2003. *La Formación del Estado y la Nación, y el Pueblo Mapuche. De la Inclusión a la Exclusión*. Santiago: Centro de Investigaciones Diego Barros Arana (Dibam).

Plancke, C. 2014. "Affect, Creativity, and Community-Making in a Congolese Song-Dance Performance: Or How to Follow the Movement of the Social." *Journal of the Royal Anthropological Institute*, 20(4): 653–69.

Polit, K. 2007. "Social Consequences of Ritual Failure: a Garhwali Case Study." In *When Rituals Go Wrong: Mistakes, Failures and the Dynamics of Ritual*, ed. U. Hüsken, 199–207. Leiden: Brill.

Pozo, G., and M. Canio. (2014). *Wenumapu: Astronomía y Cosmología Mapuche*. Santiago: Ocholibros editores.

Rappaport, J. 1994. *Cumbe Reborn: An Andean Ethnography of History*. Chicago, London: University of Chicago Press.

Richards, P. 2013. *Race and the Chilean Miracle: Neoliberalism, Democracy, and Indigenous Rights*. Pittsburgh: University of Pittsburgh Press.

Rodríguez, J.M., and J. Quidel. 2016. "Discusión sobre la Presencia de la Brujería Europea y del Chamanismo Mapuche en un Relato de Marta Brunet." *Acta Literaria*, 53: 127–53.

Salmon, A. 2010. "Aboriginal Mothering, FASD Prevention and the Contestations of Neoliberal Citizenship." *Critical Public Health*, 21(2): 165–78.

Sartre, J.P. 2004. *The Imaginary*. New York, London: Routledge.

Schechner, R. 2002. *Performance Studies: An Introduction*. London: Routledge.

Scheper-Hughes, N., and M. Lock. (1987). "The Mindful Body: A Prolegomenon to Future Work in Medical Anthropology." *Medical Anthropology Quarterly*, 1(1): 6–41.

Schieffelin, E. 1996. "On Failure and Performance: Throwing the Medium out of the Séance." In *The Performance of Healing*, ed. C. Laderman and M. Roseman, 59–89. London: Routledge.

Schieffelin, E. 2007. "Introduction." In *When Rituals go Wrong: Mistakes, Failure and the Dynamics of Ritual*, ed. U. Husken, 1–20. Leiden, Boston: Brill.

Seligman, A., P. Weller, M. Puett, and B. Simon. 2008. *Ritual and its Consequences: An Essay on the Limits of Sincerity*. Oxford: Oxford University Press.

Seremetakis, N. 1998." Durations of Pain: A Genealogy of Pain." In *Identities in Pain*, ed. J. Frykman, N. Seremetakis and S. Ewert, 151–68. Lund: Nordic Academic Press.

Singer, M. 1986. "Toward a Political-Economy of Alcoholism: The Missing Link in the Anthropology of Drinking." *Social Science & Medicine*, 23(2): 113–30.

Stolberg, M. 2015. *Uroscopy in Early Modern Europe*. Farnham: Ashgate.

Stroeken, K. 2008. "Sensory Shifts and 'Synaesthetics' in Sukuma Healing." *Ethnos*, 73(4)L 466–84.

Taussig, M. 1986. *Shamanism, Colonialism, and the Wild Man: A Study in Terror and Healing*. Chicago: University of Chicago Press.

Turner, V. 1967. "A Ndembu Doctor in Practice." In *The Forest of Symbols*, ed. V. Turner, 359–93. Ithaca: Cornell University Press.

Turner, V. 1977. *The Ritual Process: Structure and Anti-structure*. Ithaca: Cornell University Press.

Vargas, J.L. 2018. "(Galvarino) Organizaciones Mapuche Resguardan Centro de Salud Mapuche Ante Usurpación Municipal." Radio Kurruf, [online]. Retrieved 4 December 2019 from https://radiokurruf.org/2018/02/13/galvarino-organizaciones-mapuche-resguardan-centro.

Villalobos, S. 1995. *Vida Fronteriza en la Araucanía: El Mito de la Guerra de Arauco*. Santiago: Editorial Andrés Bello.

Villalobos, S. 2000. "Araucanía: Errores Ancestrales." El Mercurio, [online] A2. Retrieved 9 January 2020 from www.mapuche.info/news01/merc000606.html.

Viveiros de Castro, E. 2004. "Perspectival Anthropology and the Method of Controlled Equivocation." *Journal of the Society for the Anthropology of Lowland South America*, 2(1): 3–22.

Voss, E. 2011. "The Struggle for Sovereignty: The Interpretation of Bodily Experiences in Anthropology and Among Mediumistic Healers in Germany." In *Encounters of Body and Soul in Contemporary Religious Practices: Anthropological Reflections*, ed. R. Blanes and A. Fedele, 168–78. Oxford, New York: Berghahn.

Waitzkin, H. 1991. *The Politics of Medical Encounters: How Patients and Doctors Deal with Social Problems*. New Haven: Yale University Press.

Waldram, J.B. 2000. "The Efficacy of Traditional Medicine: Current Theoretical and Methodological Issues." *Medical Anthropology Quarterly*, 14(4): 603–25.

Waldram, J.B. 2004. *Revenge of the Windigo: The Construction of the Mind and Mental Health of North American Aboriginal Peoples*. Toronto: University of Toronto Press.

Whyte, S. 1997. *Questioning Misfortune: The Pragmatics of Uncertainty in Eastern Uganda*. Cambridge: Cambridge University Press.
Zapater, H. 1998. *Aborígenes Chilenos a Través de Cronistas y Viajeros*. Santiago: Editorial Andrés Bello.

Index